Advance Praise for
The Latino Patient

"Dr. Chong has gathered an impressive compendium of useful and relevant information in a humanized approach to caring for the Latino patient. With the wisdom of her own experiences, Dr. Chong calls the medical world to task in providing effective, culturally competent...treatment. I highly recommend this outstanding resource."

—Lourdes Baezconde-Garbanati PhD, MPH
Assistant Professor in Preventive Medicine,
W. M. Keck School of Medicine,
Institute for Health Promotion and Disease Prevention Research,
University of Southern California;
Community Outreach and Education Director,
Hispanic/Latino Tobacco Education Network and
Southern California Partnership Program Office, Cancer Information Service

"The Latino Patient *is a very lucid summary of the principles of cultural competence that should be understood by every health care provider who serves Latino patients. Dr. Nilda Chong has distilled her years of experience in working with these patients to produce a work that is both informative and a pleasure to read.*"

—Mohammad N. Akhter, MD, MPH
Executive Director, American Public Health Association

"Nilda Chong has written a highly readable, practical guide that tells non-Latino health care professionals exactly what they need to know to have effective, meaningful relationships with their Latino patients. Reading this book has enhanced my appreciation of Latino culture and made me a better doctor."

"[Considering] the very large number of Latinos living in the U.S. and the all-too-few Latino health providers available, it is a given that the vast number of Latinos in the U.S. will be cared for by non-Latino health providers. Dr. Chong has written a concise yet comprehensive book to help non-Latinos serve Latino patients more effectively and achieve better compliance. In fact, her message is worthwhile in terms of how we should treat all of our clients—with dignity, concern and compassion. I highly recommend The Latino Patient: A Guide for Health Care Providers."

"Nilda Chong has captured the essence of cross-cultural communication with Latino patients in the United States. When I was reading The Latino Patient, it felt like my family, my traditions, and my understanding of my culture were being explained to non-Latino physicians in a clear, respectful, and concise way. Nilda has taken a difficult concept and explained it in a way that is easy to comprehend and use, providing multiple examples and vignettes to address each point."

"The Latino Patient *offers clinicians a pathway toward providing culturally competent care to the fastest growing population in the country.*"

—Guadalupe Pacheco, Public Health Advisor
U.S. Department of Health and Human Services

"*In* The Latino Patient, *Dr. Chong bestows upon the reader her years of experience and wisdom in navigating the often complex interaction between Latinos and the health care system. Combining medically relevant background information, current research models and illustrative clinical vignettes,* The Latino Patient *serves as a valuable skills-building and reference tool for health care practitioners and support staff.*"

—Jeffrey R. Conly, Second-Year Medical Student
Temple University School of Medicine, Philadelphia
Former National Subcommittee Chair, American Medical Students Association

"The Latino Patient *gives health care workers a bird's-eye view of the Latino community from many angles. The overall message is clear: How can you effectively treat patients unless you have some understanding of their beliefs and desires? Amazingly, the principles of cultural understanding laid out in this book can be employed by health care workers to better serve* all *communities, a focus that is severely lacking in the American health care landscape today.*"

—Richard Cano, Second-Year Medical Student
Stanford University School of Medicine
National Co-coordinator for the Minority Affairs Committee of the
American Medical Students Association

THE Latino Patient

INTERCULTURAL PRESS
A Nicholas Brealey Publishing Company

BOSTON • LONDON

THE Latino Patient

A Cultural Guide
for
Health Care Providers

Nilda Chong
MD, DrPH

First published by Intercultural Press. For information contact:

Intercultural Press, Inc.
A division of
Nicholas Brealey Publishing
100 City Hall Plaza, Suite 501
Boston, MA 02108 USA
Tel: (+) 617-523-3801
Fax: (+) 617-523-3708
www.interculturalpress.com

Nicholas Brealey Publishing
3-5 Spafield Street
Clerkenwell
London, EC1R 4QB, UK
Tel: (+) 44-207-239-0360
Fax: (+) 44-207-239-0370
www.nicholasbrealey.com

© 2002 by Nilda Chong

Printed in the United States of America

10 09 08 07 06   3 4 5 6 7

Library of Congress Cataloging-in-Publication Data

Chong, Nilda.
    The Latino patient: a cultural guide for health care providers/
Nilda Chong.
        p. cm.
    Includes bibliographical references.
    ISBN: 1-877864-95-1 (alk. paper)
    1. Hispanic Americans—Health and hygiene. 2. Hispanic Ameri-
cans—Medical care. 3. Medical care—Cross-cultural studies. 4.
Medical care—Utilization.   I. Title.
RA448.5.H57 C56 2002
362.1'089'68073—dc21   2002068514

To Kyn,
who encouraged me to dream
about finding a way to impact Latino health
and nurtured the vision of this book
from its early beginnings.

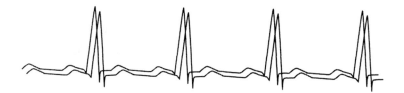

Table of Contents

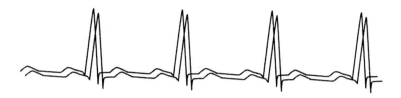

Preface

October 31, 1979

It was six in the evening; crickets were starting to chirp, and it was getting dark. The peasant woman was sweating heavily after having walked barefoot, carrying her baby son in her arms, for more than six hours. She timidly approached one of the doctors at the temporary clinic. In a single day the medical team had provided immunizations and medical and dental attention to more than five hundred people of San Juan de Dios, a community embedded in the heart of the Latin American tropical rain forest.

"Doctor," she said, "could you please see my child? He has been coughing for days. I left this morning at four o'clock but was unable to get here on time because the river near our village had overflowed. I waited two hours until the water was calm enough so that I could swim across with my baby in my arms in order to get here."

The medical team was exhausted; almost everyone was in the jeeps, and all of the medical equipment and supplies had already been packed away. They had a six-hour ride ahead of them to get back to civilization. The doctor looked at her colleagues, hesitated for a moment, and thought, "If I agree to see your child, more people are going to ask the same thing. Besides, we're all tired and everyone in the team wants to go back." The chief of the team stepped in and, addressing the peasant woman, said, "We'll see everyone that hasn't been taken care of, even if we have to leave in the middle of the night." The team leader led the doctor away from the group and explained, "Can you just imagine how big an effort this woman had to make to get here, to get the courage to approach you, a doctor, and ask for help knowing that she might get a negative answer?" The doctor had never thought about these issues before because she was an outsider and she could not relate to this community or to this woman's suffering. She could hardly relate to the ways of simple people she would probably never see again. But the experience changed her life forever. I am this doctor.

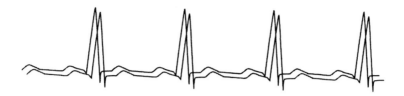

Acknowledgments

My father, Cecilio, is Chinese and my mother, Eva, is Latina. I was born and raised in Panama, a country where multiculturalism is a way of life. My parents gave me the opportunity to be who I am, a bilingual and bicultural Latina. My brothers Alvaro and Daniel were my accomplices in our early explorations of our cultural heritage.

I am convinced that the idea for this book was planted in my mind more than twenty years ago when Dr. Eyda Mariela Garrido opened the door toward my journey into cultural awareness. That was back in 1978, the year I spent working as a medical intern in the tropical rain forest of Panama. During the next twenty years, frequent colloquia with Dr. Frank Guelfi revolved around our patients' behavior and fueled my already heightened interest in cultural sensitivity toward individuals whose worlds seemed to be so distant from ours. I was often awed at the fact that, as our understanding of our patients' cultures increased, the distance between us diminished exponentially.

With humor and a keen eye, Vielka Chang-Yau influenced my work over many years, often highlighting fine distinctions between the Latino and the Chinese cultures. In the late 1980s and 1990s, Dr. Hugo Prado, Dr. Yanuario Garcia, and Francisco Castro were instrumental in shedding light on my experiences with the Pan American Health Organization/World Health Organization. Thanks to them, my work throughout Latin American countries became an exploration of Latino diversity. With the guidance of Drs. Ana and Manuel Palau, I became more aware of Latino cultural nuances that emerge within and outside of the context of the clinical encounter.

When I became a Latina immigrant, Frances Saunders inspired me to seek my truth with an honest heart and a humble mind. Dr. Lourdes Baezconde-Garbanati's love for our culture led me to embrace the commitment to participate actively in helping to improve Latino health.

During my doctoral studies at the University of California at Berkeley, Dr. Robert Hosang, Dr. Denise Herd, Dr. Lorraine Midanik, Dr. Patricia Morgan, Dr. Sylvia Guendelman, Jean Morton, Dr. Richard Stephens, and Dr. Larry Wallack were my guides. Drs. Meredith Minkler, Kurt Organista, and Eugene Garcia were instrumental in supporting my work around

Latino cultural values. Dr. Te-Wei Hu continues to support my commitment to make a contribution to American society.

Dr. Vernon Edwards and Afroze Edwards shared valuable and unique insights, often reminding me that there is a clear path toward effective communication despite cultural differences. Conversations with Javier Illueca, Sylvia Jimenez, and Dr. Maria Nieves Diaz helped me gain cultural self-awareness and figure out where to place several pieces of the puzzle. Dr. Lynette Charity shared thoughts that helped me reflect about being a person of color in a multicultural society. Allen and Linda Craig pointed out nuances of the mainstream culture that allowed me to identify aspects of intercultural communication that are addressed in several of the vignettes in this book.

I am indebted to the distinguished academics, researchers, and health professionals who reviewed this book: Guadalupe Pacheco, Jeff Conly, Richard Cano, and Drs. Terry Stein, Adriana Linares, Mohammad Akhter, Lourdes Baezconde-Garbanati, and Fernando Treviño.

In the final stages of this project, I joined Kaiser Permanente. Ron Knox's vision of diversity gave me a perspective of the Latino culture from a collective vantage point. Gayle Tang, Andrea Roberts, Sue Tico, Carlos Vargas, Roland Wilson, Jenelle Flewellen, Thuy Nguyen, and Meiska Scott reminded me every day that intercultural communication is about sharing big and small experiences.

Toby Frank, Judy Carl-Hendrick, and Stephanie

Cheney at Intercultural Press were a dream team to work with. The depth and breadth of *The Latino Patient* is, to a large extent, a result of their suggestions. I have enjoyed the experience beyond words.

To all, I gratefully express my appreciation for giving me the privilege to put in writing the products of our discussions and interactions.

—Nilda Chong, MD, DrPH, MPH
Pine Mountain Lake
Groveland, California
2002

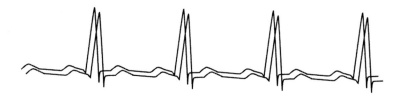

Introduction

Latinos are dramatically changing the demographic profile of the United States. They currently comprise 13.3 percent of the total population and will likely grow to roughly 20 percent in 2030 and 25 percent by 2050. Two factors help explain the Latino population boom. First, Latinas have the highest birthrate in the country for women of childbearing age. Second, every year an estimated 500,000 documented and 500,000 undocumented Latinos enter the U.S. Unfortunately, the number of Latinos in the health care workforce is proportionately much smaller than the size of the community warrants. For example, in California, where *one in three persons* were Latino, less than 5 percent of physicians were Latino in 1999 (Bureau of the Census 2001; Alcalay et al. 1992; Hayes-Bautista 1997).

Health care providers are facing the increasing demands of the thirty-five million Latinos living in the United States. Providing culturally competent care to them, that is, understanding the Latino culture in order to establish sensitive and effective communication with them during the clinical encounter, is critical for non-Latino health practitioners.

Acknowledging that culture and language may act as barriers between Latino patients and their providers, health care organizations have taken steps to develop the cultural competence of providers and to manage language issues with the help of medical interpreters. Yet, within the physician-patient relationship, cultural issues remain a gray area from the practitioners' perspective.

How can a non-Latino health care provider communicate effectively with a Latino patient? This book offers clinicians a bridge to understanding the Latino patient through a practice-based approach. For this purpose, I use vignettes that focus on common situations to illustrate a culturally oriented approach and to address difficulties in communication. By understanding the critical cultural values that differentiate the Latino patient's culture from the provider's mainstream culture and by learning some strategies for interacting in a culturally respectful manner, clinicians will be able to develop cultural competence with Latino patients.

The Latino Patient combines current cultural knowledge and key health data about Latinos with the author's personal experience of twenty years working with Latino patients in Latin America. The first part of the book defines Latino patients, their health status and attitudes, beliefs, and practices. In addition, it suggests strategies for enhancing communication and increasing sensitivity with Latino patients. The second part of the book, chapters 6 through 10, presents the author's four-step Latino Culturally Competent Care Model: GREET, LISTEN, CARE, and TREAT. Each segment of the model is designed to assist providers in their work. Reading the book as it is presented, Part I first and then Part II, is highly recommended.

Chapter 1 defines the Latino patient, presents an overview of Latino diversity, and describes the health status of U.S. Latinos. The chapter also presents the explanatory models for morbidity and mortality rates among Latinos and emphasizes the importance of culture, acculturation, and health.

Chapter 2 lists and discusses the cultural values that are most relevant to developing an effective patient-provider relationship with a Latino patient.

Chapter 3 describes Latinos' health attitudes, beliefs, and practices and their health-seeking behavior.

Chapter 4 explains how to communicate effectively with the Latino patient, how to deliver culturally appropriate health messages, and what the key elements are to help the Latino patient to adopt healthier habits.

Chapter 5 explores the concept of cultural competence and offers a self-assessment tool for providers who may want to have a general idea of their effectiveness with Latino patients. The chapter ends with a list of Dos and Don'ts with the Latino patient.

Chapter 6, "GREET: Characterizing Your Latino Patient," presents an acronym, the letters of which represent the key elements for the provider to keep in mind when first meeting a Latino patient.

Chapter 7, "LISTEN: Gaining Access to Your Patient's Clinical History," describes six key elements for enhancing communication during the history-taking interview in order to access valuable information. The chapter also describes issues that arise while dealing with the medical history as well as Latinos' common descriptions and terms for symptoms and signs.

Chapter 8 describes CARE, four key approaches to performing a culturally sensitive patient evaluation. In addition the chapter explains issues that arise during the physical exam of Latino patients with consideration of age and gender groups.

Chapter 9, "TREAT: Providing Culturally Competent Treatment," suggests ways to provide effective treatment by building trust and rapport through communication. The chapter suggests ways to recommend a treatment plan, prescribe medication, and negotiate consent for diagnostic and surgical procedures.

Chapter 10 rounds out the book with a discussion of key factors to consider in developing patient loyalty and suggests an effective farewell procedure.

Understanding that every health practitioner's personal communication style is a key element in the clinical setting, the author hopes that providers will find the suggestions offered in this book useful during their encounters with Latino patients and that each provider can find ways to adapt this material to fit his or her unique style. The author takes full responsibility for the personal contributions made in Part II.

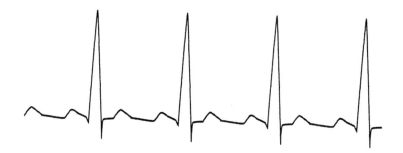

Part I
Defining the Latino Patient

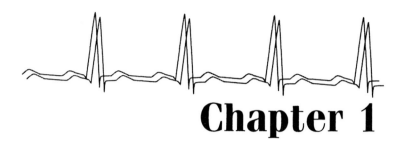

Chapter 1

Defining the Latino Patient

Who Are Latinos? Snapshot of a Diverse Population

Latinos[1] are the 35.3 million persons living in the United States who trace their origins to Latin America. In 2002 they represent about 13 percent of the total population of the U.S. and are the nation's largest mi-

---

[1] *Latino*, rather than *Hispanic*, is the term that persons who trace their origins to Latin America use to self-describe, so this is the term I will use. Latin America includes all of the nations south of the United States where Spanish is the national language, plus Brazil.

nority. The states with the highest concentration of
Latinos are California, Texas, New York, Florida, Illi-
nois, Arizona, and New Jersey (Guzmán 2001; Therrien
and Ramirez 2000; Grieco and Cassidy 2001).

With a median age of 25.9 years, Latinos are a relatively young population (the median age for the U.S.
population overall is 35 years). According to the 2000
census, 58 percent of the nation's Latinos are of Mexican origin, 10 percent are from Puerto Rico, 3.5 percent are of Cuban origin, and the remaining 28.5 percent are Central and South American, Dominican, and
of other Hispanic origins.[2]

The growth of the Latino population in the United
States is, as mentioned in the Introduction but worth
repeating here, a consequence of high birthrates and
immigration. By 2100, there will be about 190 million
Latinos living in the U.S. (Alcalay et al. 1992; Bureau
of the Census 2001).

Latinos present three challenges to health care providers: *language, diversity,* and *culture* (Trueba 1999; Chase
and Chase 1998; Gonzalez-Lee and Simon 1990; Goldsmith 1990). Language will not be discussed in depth
in this book, but diversity and culture will. Bridging
the communication gap entails having some proficiency in the Spanish language, possessing a sound
knowledge of the diversity within the Latino group,
and understanding the Latino culture. A solid knowl-

---

[2] Their poverty rate declined from 26 percent in 1998 to 21
percent in 2000. In 2001 57 percent of Latinos age 25 and
over had a high school degree and 11 percent had a bachelor's
degree (Guzmán 2001; Bureau of the Census 2001).

edge of the health needs of the various generations of this population also enhances the effectiveness of health care providers. Today non-Latino health care providers face communication and cultural barriers with Latino patients that can affect health care access (*One America* 1998).

Latino versus Hispanic

In the 1960s the U.S. Census Bureau used the term *Hispanic* to refer to persons whose native language was Spanish and/or who had Spanish ancestry (from Spain). Over the next twenty years people from Latin American countries (Mexico, Central and South America, Puerto Rico, Cuba, and the Dominican Republic) continued to immigrate and developed into the three major groups: Mexican Americans, Cuban Americans, and Puerto Ricans. The massive influx of Central Americans completed the mosaic of U.S. Latinos in the 1980s. People whose family origins were in Latin America identified themselves as *Latino* in spite of the persistent use of *Hispanic* at the governmental level. By 1993 the Census Bureau recognized the need to revisit the term *Hispanic* (Bureau of the Census 1993). Consequently, in 1996 the Census Bureau redefined *Hispanic*, and in 1997 the Office of Management and Budget issued a standard by which the terms *Latino* and *Hispanic* were to be used interchangeably. The measure is to be fully implemented by January 1, 2003 (Office of Management and Budget 1997). *Latinos*, then, is a plural noun that generically describes both men and women. However, when referring specifically to a female, the most appropriate term is *Latina*; if more than one, the term is *Latinas*. Likewise, when referring to a male or people in general, the correct term is *Latino*, or if several, *Latinos*.

Latino Diversity

Latino diversity includes social and demographic factors (Kent 1997; Council on Scientific Affairs 1991). Six of these factors are especially important for the health care provider: language, nationality, religion, race, social class, and age. They are discussed in the next sections.

Language

Spanish unites Latinos and is spoken with as many different accents and intonations as there are Spanish-speaking countries in Latin America. People from every country and region in Latin America use distinctive idiomatic speech patterns (Stoneman 1997; Council on Scientific Affairs 1991). For example, Mexicans tend to speak using a great many idioms; Central Americans' Spanish is fast-paced; and South American Spanish speakers are known for their almost musical intonations and a more educated vocabulary. Brazil is the only country in Latin America where people speak Portuguese and not Spanish.[3] Because Portuguese is

---

[3] There are also three countries in South America that are not considered part of Latin America: Suriname, Guyana, and French Guiana.

similar to Spanish, Brazilians learn it easily, so language has not been a barrier for them in communicating with other Latinos. The large number of Spanish variations among Latinos seems to have been overcome by the Latino media use of "broadcast Spanish," a form of neutral Spanish where words are pronounced without an identifiable accent and regional or national idiomatic expressions are almost entirely absent.

For providers, a basic knowledge of Spanish is highly desirable for verbal communication, but it is not absolutely required. The complexities and richness of the Spanish language add to the difficulties of developing proficiency. For those who pale at the prospect of trying to learn a foreign language, alternatives exist and more are being developed to assist providers with the language issue. Health care organizations are using translation/interpretation services, and some are enlisting medical interpreters as members of the health team (Hornberger et al. 1997). Medical interpreters must, however, be aware of regional and national expressions and idiomatic language used to describe names of ailments, symptoms, signs, and health practices. As the training and certification process of medical interpretation continues to evolve, providers may gain more by focusing on the factors that they can more easily learn in order to establish effective communication with a Latino patient. Developing cultural sensitivity is more easily attainable than is linguistic proficiency.

Nationality

In 2000, 39 percent of the Latino population (almost 13 million persons) was foreign born (Therrien and Ramirez 2000). Latinos can trace their origins to twenty-two different countries, and many immigrants from Latin America are children of immigrants themselves; for example, Brazil and Peru had significant Japanese migrations between 1899 and 1908 (Gardiner 1975), and Argentina and Chile became home to Spanish, English, German, and Italian immigrants beginning in the late nineteenth century (Levene 1937).

Latinos in the United States continue to become an even more diverse group as individuals from subgroups continue to intermarry and give rise to new generations of Latinos with mixed heritage. The differences among people from the same country can affect their health status as well. The first wave of Cubans who arrived in this country in the 1960s consisted mostly of middle- and upper-class families who had attained some level of education. In contrast, the second wave of Cubans who arrived, called the *Marielitos* because they left in boats from the Port of Mariel, were less educated and exhibited social and health problems that the prior group did not. Central Americans brought with them problems resulting from their war experiences, such as post-traumatic stress syndrome. Also many must hold more than one job in order to support family members that stayed back home. For example, approximately 20 percent of the economy of El Salvador depends on the monetary support that comes from relatives living in the U.S.

Religion

Most Latinos are Catholics. This is a consequence of the presence of Spanish conquerors who, from 1492, initiated the conversion of the natives to Catholicism. Still, people from Latin America profess all world religions, and it is not unusual to encounter Jews, Muslims, Protestants, Jehovah's Witnesses, Mormons, or Buddhists.

Religion, regardless of creed or denomination, plays a very important role in most Latinos' lives. Culturally, they focus more on the spiritual than on the material aspects of life. Also, some Latinos have combined religious beliefs with social traditions. For example, Catholics celebrate their daughters' fifteenth birthday, her coming of age, with a family party and a mass.

The attitude toward health and disease is closely linked to the perception of religion. Catholics, for instance, consider God the giver of all, including health; therefore, health is a consequence of being good, and disease may represent punishment for bad deeds. This fatalistic attitude may present a challenge for providers.

Race

The people of Latin America are a mixture of many racial groups. Latin America was visited by English, French, Portuguese, Dutch, and Spanish expeditions during the sixteenth century. From 1492 Spanish conquerors succeeded in establishing permanent roots in the New World. Later, some Latin American countries received migratory waves from Africa, Asia, and Europe. While

all races exist in Latin American countries, the makeup
of the various groups differs remarkably. For example,
Mexico's population is 60 percent mestizo (mixed European and native Indian), 30 percent Amerindian (native Indian), 9 percent white, and 1 percent other.
Guatemala's population is 56 percent mestizo and 44
percent Amerindian. The Central American country of
Costa Rica and the South American countries of Argentina, Chile, and Uruguay have predominantly white
populations. On the Caribbean islands of Cuba, the Dominican Republic/Haiti, and Puerto Rico, mulattoes
(mixed African and European) predominate.

Social Class

Closely linked with racial background is the concept
of social class in Latin America. Social class does not
appear to be a significant issue in the United States,
but it is still very much a reality for many persons of
Latin American origin. In many of the Latin American
countries, a small group of families with Spanish heritage consider themselves the founding families of the
countries and, through political and family alliances,
have maintained control of financial empires based on
businesses and vast land holdings. This upper class is,
for the most part, educated and white. Middle-class
Latin Americans are mostly the product of migratory
waves to Central and South America and therefore
range from whites to mestizos, mulattoes, and all possible combinations of racial and ethnic groupings.
Many have taken advantage of education to attain some
upward mobility. Amerindian and black groups have

historically had less access to education and economic opportunities; they are generally considered the lower class in Latin America. Fortunately, while Latinos in the U.S. are of all racial and ethnic combinations, their ancestry does not correspond to social class in this country.

Age

U.S. Latinos are a relatively young population. In 2000, 36 percent were under eighteen, 59 percent were from 19 to 65 years of age, and just over 5 percent were 65 and older. This population distribution contrasts sharply with the age distribution of the population as a whole. As the population of the United States ages, Latinos seem to be contributing to a large segment of the younger generations. It is estimated that in 2015, 25 percent of U.S. teenagers will be Latinos. Therefore, the health needs of this population present an increasing demand for preventive and curative services that are typical of young populations (Therrien and Ramirez 2000; Bureau of the Census 2001). The six factors described in this section have important public health implications that will be described in the next section.

Health Status of the
U.S. Latino Population

There is insufficient data about and a limited understanding of the health outcomes of Latinos. The 1992 report to Congress by the General Accounting Office stated, "The health status of Hispanics, especially Hispanic subgroups, is imprecisely known and [has] thus far been insufficiently analyzed. As a result, a comprehensive view of the morbidity and mortality trends of different Hispanic groups is not available at this time." Similarly, only limited data regarding the health practices and use of health services of Latinos is available (Goldsmith 1993; Council on Scientific Affairs 1991).

Despite the lack of sufficient national data, some facts are known.

1. The life expectancy of the Latino population is 79 years compared with 75 for the total population.
2. Researchers have reported improvements in infant mortality rates among certain Latino subgroups.
3. The prevalence of smoking among adults is lower, and there are increases in breast cancer screenings among women.
4. Key areas of concern about Latinos' health include prevention of diabetes, adolescent pregnancy, tuberculosis, HIV infection, violence, and obesity.
5. Increasing access to primary care services remains a challenge (Delgado 1998).

In an attempt to find explanations for Latino health outcomes, scholars have raised important issues that highlight the incongruities between Latinos' socioeconomic conditions and the health profile of this population. Two explanatory models for the Latino health profile are the *epidemiological paradox* and the *healthy migrant effect*, which are discussed in the next section.

Explaining the Latino Health Profile

The Epidemiological Paradox: The term *epidemiological para-dox* was coined by Marvin Karno and Robert Edgerton in 1969 to describe the apparent lack of correlation between the socioeconomic profile of Latinos and their health outcomes. What this means is that in spite of negative factors that would be expected to impact Latinos' health, the health profile of the group appears to be unaffected (Markides and Coreil 1986; Karno and Edgerton 1969).

Demographic, cultural, and socioeconomic factors as well as the level of acculturation have an impact on Latino health status (Alcalay et al. 1992; Sorlie et al. 1993; Muñoz 1988). The barriers they face in accessing health care negatively influence their health status, as does their acquisition of the unhealthy habits of the dominant culture. Nonetheless, Latinos' health outcomes are *much better than expected;* hence the paradox.

The Healthy Migrant Effect: Another surprise to research-ers is that Latinos not born in the United States have lower mortality rates than Latinos born here. In other words, new immigrants to the U.S. appear to be healthier and more productive than they would be expected to be (Furiño and Muñoz 1991; Sorlie et al.).

Health Facts

Morbidity

Latinos' major health problems are similar to those of the general population (Quinn and McNabb 1999;

Valdez and Narayan 1999; Delgado 1998). They include the following:

⇒ diabetes

⇒ tuberculosis

⇒ HIV infection

⇒ violence

⇒ end-state renal disease

⇒ gallbladder disease

⇒ cardiovascular diseases (coronary and ischemic heart disease, hypertension, cerebrovascular disease)

Children: The lack of access to primary care appears to characterize childhood health. Repeated ear infection, repeated tonsillitis, and pneumonia are the most common infectious illnesses. Chronic illnesses are also of concern: asthma, bronchitis, and elevated levels of lead in the blood. In addition, Latino children have low compliance rates with immunization series; consume less-than-recommended servings of bread, fruits, and vegetables; have iron intakes lower than the recommended levels; and consume more than the recommended daily cholesterol. With respect to safety, one in ten Latino children have, according to reports, an accident, injury, or poisoning event during their childhood (Delgado 1998).

Adolescents: Adolescent Latinos' health is characterized by a lack of exercise, unprotected sexual activity, abuse of alcohol and other drugs, suicide attempts, and increasing violence.

Adults: The most prevalent chronic conditions among Latino adults are heart disease, cancer, diabetes, and liver disease.

In sum, the diseases that affect the health of Latinos can be addressed by culturally competent health providers who focus on primary care and health promotion interventions.

Mortality

Latinos have higher poverty rates, lower educational attainment, and less health insurance coverage than non-Latino white Americans. Studies have found that the lower socioeconomic levels are related to poor health expressed as morbidity and mortality rates. Even so, several studies have revealed "lower income-adjusted mortality rates for cancer, cardiovascular disease, and all-cause mortality among Latinos relative to non-Latino whites" (Liao et al. 1998; Sorlie et al. 1993). Therefore, it appears that the paradox holds for Latino mortality as well as morbidity.

The healthy migrant effect and the salmon bias effect[4] have been used to explain the low mortality rates of Latinos. Some researchers have posited that the healthy migrant effect might explain the lower mortality rates among Latinos. They suggest that Latinos who immigrate to the United States are healthier individuals and therefore have lower mortality rates than those of Latinos who remain in their homeland (Sorlie et al.; Furiño and Muñoz; Shai and Rosenwaike 1987). Other researchers have attributed

---

[4] Wishing to die in their own birthplace, "...many Latinos return to their countries of birth after temporary employment, retirement, or becoming seriously ill" (Herrera et al. 1994). This is known as the "salmon bias" effect.

this phenomenon to the salmon bias effect (Abraido-Lanza et al. 1999; Pablos-Mendez 1994). Yet, neither of the two hypotheses explains the mortality epidemiological paradox. Some researchers even suggest that "better health practices, especially relative to risk factors for heart disease and cancer," might explain the lower mortality rates. If that were the case, however, then there would not be an epidemiological paradox (1999). Clearly, more research is needed.

According to the U.S. Census Bureau (2000), the ten leading causes of death for Latinos of both sexes and all ages, in rank order, are

1. diseases of the heart,
2. malignant neoplasms,
3. accidents,
4. cerebrovascular disease,
5. diabetes mellitus,
6. pneumonia and influenza,
7. homicide and legal intervention,
8. chronic liver disease and cirrhosis,
9. chronic obstructive pulmonary disease, and
10. certain conditions originating in the perinatal period.

Factors in the Decision to Seek Health Care

This section describes factors that may impact the decision to seek health care: language, health insurance coverage, and acculturation. As already discussed (see pages 6–7), language can act as a critical barrier to Latino access to health care services, so I won't belabor the point here.

Health Insurance Coverage

Although Latinos are the most highly employed minority and almost two-thirds have health insurance coverage, that still leaves more than one-third without basic coverage. In contrast, only 15 percent of the entire American population lacks health insurance coverage (Goldsmith 1990). Mexican Americans, who make up 58 percent of all Latinos, have particularly low rates of health insurance because they are employed in the low-skilled and low-paid sectors of the economy that are less likely to provide insurance coverage to their employees as a benefit. Mexican Americans' and Puerto Ricans' low incomes also often prevent them from purchasing private health insurance coverage (General Accounting Office 1992; Ginzberg 1991). Consequently, Latinos are particularly vulnerable to slipping through the cracks in the current system of obtaining medical care (Carrasquillo et al. 2000; Berk et al. 2000; Valdez et al. 1993).

Unable to find access to adequate health care, many poor Latinos seek care in the emergency rooms of large public hospitals. While emergency rooms provide temporary solutions to their health problems, they cannot provide follow-up care or preventive services (Phillips 2000; Alcalay et al. 1992).

Acculturation

Acculturation encompasses the adjustments that individuals make in order to adapt to a new culture. For Latinos, these changes include learning to live in an environment that is saturated with rules and regulations. Habits that are second nature for Americans, such as taking a number, waiting in line, filling out forms, walking on the right side of a hallway, and so on, can be a nightmare for Latinos. The health care system in the United States might seem highly bureaucratic and even hostile to immigrant Latinos (Delgado 1998). In contrast, the health care system in Latin America is often more user-friendly because of the paternalistic and informal tone of providers. For some Latinos, the best option is to seek help from a folk healer who often gives very personalized attention.

Medicaid coverage and higher acculturation level have been positively associated with a greater probability for inpatient medical admission; however, a lower degree of acculturation accompanied by the perception of having good health may cause persons of Mexican origin to be less likely to seek outpatient medical care (Wells et al. 1989). Kyriakos Markides and Jeannine Coreil have suggested that a less acculturated lifestyle may afford some protection to Latinos' health, but more specific identification and understanding of these cultural and social factors are needed (1986). These protective social and cultural factors seem to have less impact on Latinos' health as their level of acculturation increases (Marin and Posner

1995; Palinkas 1994; Gilbert 1991; Caetaño and Mora 1988). For example, it has been suggested that exposure to the new culture, new friends, and English language media may influence immigrant Mexican women to begin drinking and smoking. Investigators have recommended that the focus of prevention programs directed at Mexican women be structured to target and respond to their differential levels of acculturation (Palinkas 1994; Gilbert 1991).

In sum, Lloyd Rogler et al. suggests, "increases in acculturation alienate the person from traditional supportive primary groups. Increased acculturation also facilitates the internalization of host-society cultural norms, among which are damaging stereotypes of prejudicial attitudes toward Hispanic people" (Rogler et al. 1991).

The current health status of Latinos is cause for optimism, provided appropriate and effective measures are undertaken to identify and treat their preventive and curative health care needs (Molina and Aguirre-Molina 1994; Vega 1994). The challenge of maintaining and, better yet, improving the Latino health profile will continue to demand more research regarding Latino health outcomes and a greater understanding of the impact of acculturation and health education on health behaviors. While increasing the number of Latino practitioners is highly desirable, developing cultural competence of non-Latino health providers remains a reasonable, effective, and attainable option to help maintain the Latino health profile.

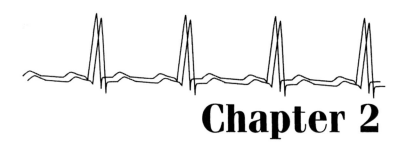

Chapter 2

Cultural Values of
the Latino Patient

Latinos are a diverse group held together by a common language and a set of cultural values. In particular, generational differences often determine the degree to which both are adhered to. First-generation immigrants generally hold fast to their culture and attempt to transmit the same values to their children. With more time in the country and with continued acculturation, individuals gradually become incorporated into mainstream society. Thus, second, third, and fourth generations increasingly mirror mainstream culture (Padilla 1980).

Regardless of the level of acculturation or generation, however, Latinos retain at least three basic value sets that differ from mainstream values. First, while the dominant culture is individualistic, Latinos are group- and family-oriented. Second, mainstream culture focuses on personal, social, and financial achievement; Latino culture seeks harmonious relationships and cooperation at almost any cost. Third, while the dominant culture derives respect from success, for Latinos, respect is a consequence of age, gender, and/or hierarchy (Lecca 1998).

A competent health care provider will want to consider these differences in order to understand a Latino patient's perspective during the clinical encounter. The attitudes and responsiveness of Latino patients may be heavily conditioned by their values. The provider must actually have two perspectives in clear view if the patient-provider encounter is to meet mutual expectations: the Latino patient's perception of mainstream culture and the provider's own cultural sensitivity to the value system of the patient. This chapter presents the most common Latino cultural characteristics that are likely to emerge in the clinical setting and highlights differences in Latino subgroups.

Various scholars have described Latino cultural values. Amado Padilla's pioneering work on Latino acculturation proposed five central Latino cultural values: familism, *simpatía* (see page 27 for an explanation), *respeto* (respect), gender issues, and time orientation (1980). Other scholars proposed adding religiosity and loyalty (Magaña and Clark 1995), and later, Gerardo Marin and Barbara Van Oss Marin contributed three more values: allocentrism, power distance, and personal space (1991).

More recently, John Kikoski and Catherine Kikoski have reviewed the literature from a managerial perspective. Their list of Latino values includes self-worth, dignity and respect, manliness, womanliness, sensitivity, honesty, hierarchy, and religiosity (1996).

Relevant Latino Cultural Values

For the purpose of the patient-provider relationship, I have chosen nine Latino cultural values that I feel have the most impact on the clinical encounter: collectivism, familism, *personalismo*, gender issues, power distance, respect, religiosity, simpatía, and time orientation. This section briefly describes these key cultural values and, whenever appropriate, compares them with mainstream values and examines the evolution of the values as a consequence of adjustments to the new culture. Most of these values will be illustrated in eight vignettes later in this chapter. They will also be woven throughout chapters 6 through 9.

Collectivism

The behavior of Latinos is permeated by collectivism. This means that Latinos prefer the company of others over being alone for personal satisfaction and for self-assurance. From the Latino perspective, the relationships shared in the social or work group give strength to the collective and provide a sense of belonging. Life is viewed, therefore, from the group perspective rather than from the typically mainstream individualistic angle. (See Vignette 1, page 30.)

Familism

The Latino family is a complex and vital social organization and includes the nuclear and extended family. Family members are closely tied together by sentiments of respect, loyalty, and unity; all members must abide by these principles without question. Although the father is the authority figure, he spends most of his time outside the house working to fulfill his duties as provider. The mother takes care of the house and the children and thus often accumulates a great deal of power. This is largely because upon coming to the United States, Latinas are required to develop new skills in carrying out their role as a mother. They find out what forms they need from public offices and learn how to complete them. They take their children to school, meet other women at the school, get groceries at the supermarket, and go to church. In sum, their tasks involve getting out of the house more often than they would in their own culture. Consequently, they often participate in community activities and develop a strong social support group (Balcazar et al. 1997; Davis and Chavez 1995; Hurtado 1995; Sabogal et al. 1987; Rueschenberg and Buriel 1989). Because family unity is "sacred" for Latinos, health issues are most effectively dealt with at the family level if possible. (See Vignette 2, page 32.)

Personalismo

Personalismo is the human quality of being able to relate on a personal level, regardless of social or financial standing. It conveys respect among peers and grants admiration or respect to all persons. Also called self-worth, personalismo is based on knowledge of a person's individual qualities, learned over years of friendship and sharing. The ability to keep one's humility despite improved financial standing is clear in the vignette on personalismo (see Vignette 3, page 33).

Gender Issues

Machismo and *marianismo* are at the forefront of Latino gender issues (Mayo 1997; Gil and Vazquez 1996). Machismo, or manliness, places the man at the center of the Latino social life. Manliness may be exhibited through courage, or even an authoritarian attitude. A man's manliness may be threatened by public embarrassment, implications of a lack of masculinity, or a woman's lack of acknowledgment for a man's position in the family or in a social group activity. Marianismo, on the other hand, refers to a woman's position in the family and at home. She is expected to be as perfect as the Virgin Mary. Women earn the respect of family and friends for their dedication to their children and husbands. Marianismo is not openly acknowledged outside the home if the husband is present; a woman's domain is the house and her children.

It must be noted that the process of acculturation reshapes gender relationships and roles as Latinas become more independent and enjoy more freedom in the United States. Consequently, the decision-making process in the family usually becomes more democratic as the acculturation process proceeds. Thus, both men and women who have been here for some time are involved in the decision to seek help for family members with regard to health-related problems (see Vignette 4, page 35).

Power Distance

Power distance, or hierarchy, involves deferential treatment toward persons perceived to be in positions of power. This attitude involves obedience on the basis of respect. The perception of hierarchy may be based on knowledge, as is the case of a Latino's perception that a physician knows more about health and disease than he or she does and therefore is automatically accorded respect. (See Vignette 5, page 37.)

Respect

For Latinos respect is a sense of admiration granted because of an intrinsic quality of the individual regardless of social, political, or financial standing. Such traits as honesty, integrity, and courage are deserving of respect. Respect may also be granted to an individual because of a hierarchical standing (power distance); subordinates normally respect a supervisor. Latinos need to perceive respect in their relationships, and a lack of this perception may be interpreted as an *absence* of respect. Initiating a relationship with a stranger, for example a health care provider, is often based on perceived respect. (See Vignette 6 page 39.)

Religiosity

Latinos have profound reverence for God and for other powerful forces they believe exist. The Virgin Mary,

saints, and angels are often invoked and asked to in-
tercede before God when a Latino is asking for help
(see Vignette 7, page 40). Latinos' religious faith is connected to their fatalistic view of life. In other words,
one must face and accept the inevitability of one's fate
because it is God's will. There is also a close link between religion and family. If a man and a woman marry
in the church, the relationship is said to be "blessed by
God." In contrast, an unmarried couple is said to be
"living in sin." Views of religion and its centrality to
life may differ between men and women. For women,
God is the first priority because He is the giver of all,
including health. In contrast, men's first priority is often health because they provide for the family and
therefore must be well enough to work. For many
Latinos, men and women alike, health and disease may
be deemed consequences of God's approval or disap-
proval of a person's behavior.

Simpatía

Simpatía implies the ability to develop a harmonious
relationship that expresses a warm and caring attitude.
It does not mean "sympathy," as its similarity to the
word would seem to imply. Individuals who have this
ability are described as *simpático* or *simpática* because they
have such people-oriented skills.

Time Orientation

Time management is not a critical issue for Latinos. In
their countries of origin, they led more relaxed lives
with less bureaucratic systems of health care. In the

United States, Latinos appear to be relaxed about time and often encounter problems budgeting time and keeping to schedules in accordance with the practices of the mainstream culture. Consequently, they are often late for appointments (Madriz 1998; Delgado 1998; Spector 1996; Marin and Marin 1991). I have observed that sometimes second- and even third-generation Latinos, when interacting with other Latinos, also appear to be relaxed about time.

A provider with knowledge and understanding of Latino cultural values holds the key to establishing culturally appropriate verbal and nonverbal communication strategies with patients. Overcoming the nonverbal communication barrier rests on developing the skills to recognize and deal with cultural issues and to create effective rapport with the Latino patient during the clinical encounter. Two vital aspects of Latino communication styles and the three most relevant nonverbal styles will be discussed next.

Latino Communication Styles and Preferences

Indirect versus Direct Styles

When dealing with uncomfortable subjects or serious health concerns, Latinos often delay asking direct questions and offer indirect responses to questions. This can be disconcerting to the provider who is used to seeing patients show up with a written list of symptoms or with Internet printouts regarding disease management.

Passive versus Active Styles

Another method that some Latinos use to avoid the difficulties of facing serious health matters, especially those that involve social issues, is to speak about the problem that others have (alcoholism, drugs, etc.) while adopting a passive role suggesting that the speaker is a mere observer of the situation that others face.

Nonverbal Behavior

Personal space and touch are important to Latinos, who communicate through physical contact and appreciate physical closeness. They often kiss, shake hands, and embrace family members and friends (Axtell 1991). A handshake is expected at the initial clinical encounter and at the end of the interview by both men and women patients. With children you may be more open and playful. For example, playfully shaking both hands of a child might help you gain some trust from the parent (see Vignette 8 on page 42 on personal space). Knowing when to make and how long to maintain eye contact with the patient is also very important. Gender issues play a significant role in eye contact, as might be expected. Appropriate distance, touch, and eye contact behavior will be brought to bear numerous times in the vignettes in Part II.

The next section presents eight vignettes to illustrate collectivism, familism, personalismo, gender issues, power distance, respect, religiosity, and nonverbal behavior. A discussion follows each vignette.

Illustrative Vignettes

The following vignettes describe clinical encounters between a first-generation Latino male patient (Mr. Pérez) and a non-Latino provider (Dr. Smith) who is trying to help the patient with his drinking problem.

Vignette 1—Collectivism

Dr. Smith:	How often do you consume alcohol, Mr. Pérez?
Mr. Pérez:	In my country we drink it, but only on weekends.
Dr. Smith:	Do you use alcohol on weekends?
Mr. Pérez:	Well, only when my friends and I get together. We do it to share.
Dr. Smith:	How often do you see your friends?
Mr. Pérez:	On Saturdays and Sundays and whenever there is a holiday.
Dr. Smith:	How much alcohol do you normally drink on weekends?
Mr. Pérez:	Not much. We mostly have beers because we try not to drink strong alcohol. Back home we used to buy beer by the bottles. Here, well, we buy it by the case! (He laughs.)
Dr. Smith:	When do you stop "sharing" on weekends?
Mr. Pérez:	When it gets late, when we run out of ammunition, or when our women come to get us. We usually meet at one of our houses so the wives know

where we are. After all, we all live in the same neighborhood. We're all friends and always take care of each other when we have drinks together.

Discussion

⇒ Although Dr. Smith asked a personal question, he did not receive a straightforward answer. Instead, Mr. Pérez' reply made reference to his group's behavior regarding alcohol use.

⇒ Dr. Smith understands that "sharing" refers to collectivism. Mr. Pérez describes drinking alcohol with his friends as an experience that all the members of the group share.

⇒ Dr. Smith notices that with the interdependence that exists among the male friends, self-control is not at issue. The issue, from the Latinos' perspective, is more related to sharing and making sure that nobody gets hurt or sick while drinking together.

⇒ Many Latinos regard alcoholic beverages according to their own scale, beer being in the lowest position. Therefore, Mr. Pérez does not see a reason for self-control. The limit to his consumption of beer seems to be set by availability and his wife's appearance to take him home.

⇒ Sharing is both an attitude and a behavior among Latinos. Men drink together and, through jokes, make light of their tribulations. The experience provides an outlet for confiding their fears, concerns, plans, and dreams to their friends.

Vignette 2—Familism

Dr. Smith: Does your wife approve of your
               drinking habits?

Mr. Pérez: Well, maybe she's not crazy about it,
               but she's never said anything. I know
               that she appreciates the fact that I
               never fail to put money on the table.

Dr. Smith: Does that mean that she doesn't
               mind?

Mr. Pérez: No, it means that she knows I'm a
               very responsible parent. She's always
               said that I'm a good father because
               my children have always had what
               they needed. Besides, I always let her
               know where I am going to be. I have
               always respected my family. I've
               never gone to a bar ever since I
               married my wife.

Discussion

⇒ Knowing that Latina wives are very resourceful, Dr.
   Smith is seeking to identify a source of support
   for Mr. Pérez. Yet, because of familism, Mr. Pérez
   perceives that his family is well taken care of and
   that he is a responsible and respectful father and
   husband.

Vignette 3—Personalismo

Dr. Smith: Why do you drink with your friends?

Mr. Pérez: We became friends when we arrived here years ago. We all helped out when one of us was in any kind of trouble. We trust each other a lot because we've known each other for years.

Dr. Smith: So why do you drink together? Is it because you are stressed-out?

Mr. Pérez: In a way we may be stressed-out from work, but we also have to celebrate that we are all still here and struggling together.

Dr. Smith: Do you and your friends also work together?

Mr. Pérez: We used to be co-workers when we first got here. That's how we met. But now everybody has a different employer. That's what makes our group even more special. None of us has changed a bit! We're still the same friends.

Discussion

⇒ While Dr. Smith is searching for an etiology of Mr. Pérez' drinking pattern, Mr. Pérez is trying to explain the reasons why he values the friendship he shares with his buddies.

⇒ Dr. Smith understands that Mr. Pérez has high regard *for* his friends and is also highly regarded *by*
his friends because of the experiences they have
shared throughout the years. Thus, pursuing this
approach will not lead to finding clues that might
explain Mr. Pérez' drinking problem.

Vignette 4—Gender Issues (Machismo and Marianismo)

Dr. Smith: Mr. Pérez, does your wife also drink beer?

Mr. Pérez: Oh, no, no. She's a decent woman. She never drinks.

Dr. Smith: Have you seen her drinking at home?

Mr. Pérez: Well, she only drinks punch or a beer or two but only during family parties or holidays. Those are special days because that's when the whole family gets together and toasts. She also drinks with her cousins when they come to visit but only on special occasions and only in the house. My wife is almost a saint. I always kid her and tell her that one day I'm going to try to get her drunk.

Dr. Smith: Does she ever drink with you at home?

Mr. Pérez: No, never. She says she prefers to know that I'm with my friends as long as I tell her where I am and we don't go to the bar. As I told you, we always go to one of the guys' houses.

Discussion

⇒ Dr. Smith's attempt to find out if Mr. Pérez' wife is also abusing alcohol is met with Mr. Pérez' view of his wife's marianismo. Mr. Pérez immediately feels the need to make clear there's no doubt regarding his wife's reputation ("My wife is almost a saint").

⇒ Drinking at a friend's house and letting the wives know where the friends are meeting is socially acceptable. Getting together to have drinks at a bar with friends is not. Bars are considered to be places where temptations may arise (e.g., meeting "indecent" women).

Vignette 5—Power Distance

Dr. Smith: Have you thought about the health
               consequences of drinking alcohol?

Mr. Pérez: No, not really. I don't know much
               about it.

Dr. Smith: Well, alcohol damages people's livers
               and can seriously hurt their mental
               states.

Mr. Pérez: I think I heard about a neighbor who
               died of cirrhosis. Is that what you're
               talking about?

Dr. Smith: That's right. The liver may become
               unable to filter the blood effectively.
               It can get as hard as a rock and fail.

Mr. Pérez: Why did my neighbor die?

Dr. Smith: His liver was not able to filter and
               clean his blood. He probably died
               poisoned with his own body's waste
               substances.

Discussion

⇒ Dr. Smith first explored Mr. Pérez' interest in learning about the health consequences of alcohol. This
  gave Dr. Smith a power differential because he had
  more knowledge.

⇒ After establishing power distance, Dr. Smith took
  the next step. He talked about the damage that
  alcohol can cause to people's (not Mr. Pérez') liver.
  This created the opportunity for Mr. Pérez to ask
  more questions.

⇒ Finally, Mr. Pérez asked the question related to death. He was indirectly confiding in Dr. Smith about his fear of dying as a consequence of his alcohol use.

⇒ Because of machismo, Latino men resent being preached to. Yet, once Mr. Pérez acknowledged a need to know, he openly expressed his health concerns.

Vignette 6—Respect

Dr. Smith: If you had the opportunity, would
              you like to try to drink less alcohol?

Mr. Pérez: Well, I don't think so. Most week-
              ends I share drinks at my boss'
              house. He is also my friend, and he
              is in charge of the crew. I respect
              him as I respect my father. He often
              invites me to his house on weekends.

Dr. Smith: Do you think that your boss might
              be a negative influence on you?

Mr. Pérez: Oh, no! He's my boss. I feel honored
              that he invites me to his house often.
              He's always telling me how much he
              respects me.

Discussion

⇒ Dr. Smith's attempts to even move toward suggesting therapy are hampered by Mr. Pérez' respect
for his boss and the perception that his boss also
respects him.

Vignette 7—Religiosity

Mr. Pérez: Dr. Smith, I came to see you six months ago. Do you remember me?

Dr. Smith: Of course I do, Mr. Pérez.

Mr. Pérez: Well, after that long talk we had, I went home and told my wife about our conversation. She told me she didn't like my drinking. I realized I had a problem with alcohol.

Dr. Smith: Did you seek help?

Mr. Pérez: Well, I had to because I hadn't realized my oldest son was also drinking. My wife said he was imitating me because I'm the man of the house.

Dr. Smith: So what happened next?

Mr. Pérez: Well, I went to church with my family. My wife made me kneel at the altar and made me promise God that I was going to stop drinking. We all cried together that day.

Dr. Smith: Did you stop drinking then?

Mr. Pérez: Well, my wife also took me to AA. She had found out about it through some of her cousins whose husbands had gone through the same experience.

Dr. Smith: When was the last time you had a drink?

Mr. Pérez: About five months ago. I owe it to God. I've asked His forgiveness. I don't want to blow this second chance He's given me. And, my wife is helping me. Now we do more things together as a family on weekends, and my boy respects me again. That's very important for me, you know? After all, he needs to learn how to be a man from me!

Discussion

⇒ Dr. Smith realizes that his low-key approach motivated Mr. Pérez to reflect about his drinking problem. By sharing his thoughts with his wife, Mr. Pérez was able to admit his problem and seek help. The communication established by Dr. Smith strengthened the provider's encounter with Mr. Pérez.

⇒ Mr. Pérez' loyalty toward Dr. Smith is evidenced in the fact that he went back to see him to acknowledge his gratitude for the doctor's help. Although the message is not directly conveyed because of machismo, Mr. Pérez obviously feels indebted to Dr. Smith.

Vignette 8—Personal Space

Dr. Smith: Mr. Pérez, I'd like to examine your abdomen. Does it hurt here?

Mr. Pérez: A little bit, it feels like there's some kind of inflammation there.

Dr. Smith: I'm going to order some laboratory tests for you, O.K.?

Mr. Pérez: O.K. I guess you have to find out if something is wrong inside, right?

Dr. Smith: That's right.

Mr. Pérez: When should I come back to see you?

Dr. Smith: Call me after you've gone to the lab, and we'll decide when you'll come back to see me. (He hands him his business card while speaking.) You'll soon be in good shape for your family. (Dr. Smith smiles, stands up and moves a few inches closer, shakes Mr. Pérez' right hand, and puts his left hand on Mr. Pérez' right forearm while making eye contact with him.)

Discussion

⇒ By decreasing personal distance, shaking hands, and making eye contact with Mr. Pérez, Dr. Smith established an effective, culturally appropriate relationship with his patient.

⇒ Mr. Pérez is setting aside his machismo when he asks Dr. Smith when the next appointment should be. In addition, he's moving toward taking personal responsibility for his health. Latinos are more accustomed to a paternalistic system of health care.

Examples of Latino Cultural Values Often Encountered during the Clinical Encounter	
Cultural Value	Behavior
Collectivism	Taking friends and/or relatives to the provider's office
Familism	Failing to reveal the existence of dysfunctional relations among family members to maintain the integrity of the family's secrets
Personalismo/ Self-worth	Expressing interest in overcoming a health problem despite all odds
Machismo	Refusing a digital rectal examination
Marianismo	Taking responsibility for the health of all family members
Power distance	Accepting the clinician's knowledgeable recommendations
Respect	Standing up until asked to sit down when the provider is a female
Religiosity	Explaining that God has kept a family member in good health
Simpatía	Bringing homemade food or a present for the provider on a subsequent visit
Time orientation	Being late and explaining that the parking lot was full
Personal space	Appreciating a health care provider's handshake or a touch on the arm when leaving the office

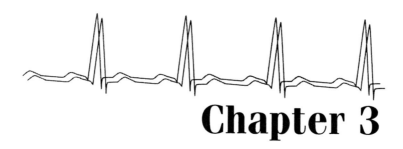

Chapter 3

Health Attitudes, Beliefs, and Practices

Historical Influences on Attitudes, Beliefs, and Practices

The roots of most Latinos' views on health and disease are found in the history of Latin America and are a combination of native Indian, African, Asian, and European influences.

Herbalists, botanists, and folk healers practiced native Indian medicine. Immigrants from Africa and Asia arrived in the Americas and also contributed their health and disease beliefs to the local culture. European conquerors brought their Hippocratic humoral theory of disease to their colonial enclaves on the American continent. According to the humoral theory of disease, or the hot and cold theory, there are four bodily humors or fluids: blood (hot and wet), yellow bile (hot and dry), phlegm (cold and wet), and black bile (cold and dry). In this model, when the four humors are balanced a person is healthy; disease is a manifestation of an imbalance. While other cultures also draw from the conceptual basis of the humoral theory, the intersection of the Latino culture and the humoral theory is uniquely manifested in the interpretation of the causes of illness and in the management of disease (Centro San Bonifacio 1997; Spector 1996).

A patient who experiences frequent bouts of nausea and who regularly vomits small amounts of a yellow fluid may attribute the problem to an upset gallbladder. Some believe that excessively fat pork may trigger secretion of large amounts of hot, yellow bile. Similarly, some Latinos consider "hot blood" as the cause of pimples that surface during adolescence.

The management of elevated body temperature, according to the humoral theory, involves offering the patient a cool drink to lower the temperature. In particular, a Latino patient's fever may be managed by offering rice or barley water to help cool the body. By the same token, the principles of the humoral theory apply to cold temperature. Drinking warm fluids can offer some help to a patient who has a cold. In the Latino culture, a bowl of hot chicken or dove soup, a hot lemonade, or hot lemongrass tea may be therapeutic measures of choice.

Other Influences on the Latino Perception of Health

Latinos describe health as "a state of well-being." The concept is so ingrained in their lives that when Latinos toast, they use the word *salud* (health) in the same manner that *cheers* is used in the United States. Despite the common denotation of the concept of health, nuances in the definition may be shaped by a number of factors including education, country of origin, generation, the number of years living in the U.S., and exposure to a different health care system prior to moving to the U.S. In fact, these influences contribute in varying combinations to particular perceptions of health among different Latino subgroups (Manzanedo et al. 1980).

Education

Educated Latinos generally subscribe to the biomedical model of health and in general would agree with the World Health Organization's definition as "a state of complete physical, mental, and social well-being and not merely the absence of disease." In contrast, those with less education might take a stance strongly influenced by the religious perspective. For them, God is, as I mentioned earlier, the giver of all, including health. Consequently, their perception of the symptoms of disease or the cause of an accident reflects their religious beliefs. Therefore, having a fractured arm as a consequence of a fall may be God's warning of future penalties for disobeying divine laws. On the other

hand, a cancer diagnosis may be God's punishment for
one's bad actions.

Country of Origin

The country of origin may also contribute to varying
views of health (New York Task Force on Immigrant
Health 1996a and 1996b). A young man who has emigrated from Guatemala, where 80 percent of the population is indigenous and rural, will probably have a traditional view of health. In contrast, a native of Argentina, a country that received a large influx of European
migration, may perceive good health as a result of having an adequate diet and a strenuous exercise regime.
Still, there is no absolute rule of thumb.

Generation

Each generation of Latinos has different health perceptions and needs that reflect their beliefs and attitudes toward health and disease. Their access to health
care services is also affected by how long they have
lived in the United States. As mentioned previously,
immigrants from Latin America began arriving in the
U.S. in large groups around the turn of the twentieth
century. Those groups are represented by several generations, and there are fewer generations of latecom-
ers. For example, although there may be as many as
three or even four generations of a Mexican American
family, there are probably still only one or two generations of Central Americans residing here.

First Generation: There are three important factors to
consider with first-generation Latinos: legal status, rea-

son for immigrating, and level of acculturation. First, having a legal right to reside in the country allows an individual to have a job and help support the family; it also provides peace of mind to pursue life in this country with ambition and hope. On the other hand, an "illegal alien" generally lives in fear of deportation, struggles with short-term low-paying jobs, and is often unwilling to provide accurate personal information out of fear of being noticed by immigration authorities.

The second consideration with first-generation immigrants involves the reasons for which they decided to move to this country. In most cases, economic, political, and social factors in their countries of origin triggered Latinos' decision to immigrate to the United States. Mexicans in search of better living conditions became the first group of Latinos to establish themselves in the U.S. at the turn of the twentieth century. In the 1960s, the first group of Cubans fled their country in the "freedom flights" when Fidel Castro turned their country toward communism. Because they fled for political reasons, they were eligible for political asylum in the U.S. The third group of Latinos to arrive in large numbers were the Central Americans who fled civil wars in Nicaragua and El Salvador. Upon arriving in the U.S., however, they were denied political refugee status. Most entered the country illegally, but many later took advantage of the moratorium offered by the Immigration and Naturalization Service and legalized their status in the country. Many, though, still live in fear of deportation. The fourth group of Latino immigrants were those

from South America. Their impact has been less significant in absolute and relative numbers, and their experience as immigrants in search of a better life has been
more positive. The fact that they were more educated
upon arrival has contributed to their being more readily
accepted into mainstream society (Repak 1994;
Hamilton and Chinchilla 1991).

Political asylum has important implications because
it allows immigrants to take advantage of governmental support that facilitates the process of finding a job,
educating their children, becoming acculturated, and
eventually becoming U.S. citizens. For example, to this
date a Cuban immigrant is still eligible to become a
U.S. citizen after a one-year stay in the country, but
the other groups must wait five years after obtaining
legal residence to become citizens.

Third, the level of acculturation, or adjustment to
the local culture, increases the diversity of the group
(Rogler et al. 1991). Acculturation may be related to
the number of years that the person has lived in the
country (although not necessarily a linear relationship)
and to the age at which the person arrived in the United
States. Elderly immigrants, for instance, face more
challenges adjusting to a new country than do younger
adults (Gelfand 1989). Many cultural values are re-
tained consciously and voluntarily, but others are modi-
fied as individuals adjust to the new country. For example, as length of time in the U.S. increases, Latinos
gradually take on the lifestyles of the mainstream culture, adopt a more permissive attitude toward alcohol
and tobacco, and consume more junk food.

Second Generation: Most second-generation Latinos grew up in a home environment that reflected their parents' country of origin. The exposure to mainstream culture at school contributed to their becoming bilingual and bicultural. As children they became their parents' interpreters with English-speaking persons. As teenagers, many felt caught between two cultures and had identity issues as their parents continued to struggle with acculturation.

Third Generation and Beyond: This group is part of mainstream society. They may call themselves Mexican Americans and Cuban Americans to express their pride in their heritage and to retain cultural values that do not conflict with the mainstream culture such as food and music. While they consider themselves bicultural, most are not proficient in Spanish; many are monolingual English speakers.

In sum, first-generation Latinos are more attached to their countries of origin, including the model of health care that they subscribed to there. Subsequent generations usually adopt the beliefs of the local mainstream culture. Adjustment to the new culture may give rise to conflicting views on health among family members of different generations. An immigrant Mexican mother may encounter difficulties when trying to explain to her second-generation daughter that she should not iron her clothes, put them on, and go out immediately; a warmed body exposed to cold weather is a call for disease. A second-generation teenager of Mexican origin who has acquired the habits of the dominant culture may find such an explanation ridiculous.

Years Living in the United States

As the years go by, Latinos increasingly embrace the biomedical model. A Cuban American woman who has lived in the United States for twenty years probably views health as most mainstream Americans do. On the other hand, a newly arrived Peruvian woman may be more attached to the magico-religious view of health of her country (or region or village) of origin.

It is also fair to state that cultural values such as familism and respect toward God often continue to strongly influence Latinos' views on health. Some Latinas believe that God is the giver of health and money (Alcalay et al. 1992; White and Maloney 1990); consequently, even second-generation adults may continue to use the home remedies their parents taught them to believe in when they were growing up. Likewise, it is not unusual to encounter educated Latinos who, while clearly understanding the biological, psychological, and social bases of health, may rate their personal health as good because of their faith in God. In fact, it is common to hear Latinos of all walks of life reflecting their religious cultural heritage by saying they have good health "thanks to God."

Prior Health Care System

Because about 36 percent of U.S. Latinos are foreign-born and because immigrant Latinos' attitudes toward health generally evolve only slowly with acculturation, it is important to examine the system of health care in which these persons lived prior to immigrating to the United States. Although the generally accepted no-tion is that Latino immigrants come from deprived systems of health care and that their health status upon arrival is in a neglected state, as we've seen that is often not the case. The health care system in Latin America is characteristically paternalistic; therefore, citizens of Latin American countries are often the beneficiaries of aggressive preventive health campaigns. In most of these countries, health services for the majority of the population are generally run by the government and operate in tandem with privately owned hospitals and outpatient clinics.

The public health sector is organized into a network of community health centers that refer patients to regional, national general, and specialized hospitals. In spite of the financial difficulties within the system, emergency services are given priority by the government to ensure their availability. Elective services, on the other hand, depend more heavily on availability of resources, and needless to say, the demand for these services usually exceeds resources.

In Latin America the health care systems strongly emphasize developing healthy lifestyles through health-promotion activities and extensive patient education programs. Through its somewhat paternalistic system of health care, each country maintains and enforces strict norms regarding child immunization, pregnancy controls, dental health, and wellness clinics for children, youth, adults, and the elderly. The health of children and youth is a priority and is promoted through school health programs supported by government agencies. Occupational safety and health programs are often provided at no charge by the ministries of health to the private and public sectors.

People who are employed have the option of using social security hospitals and clinics or seeking medical attention in private clinics and hospitals. The unemployed population is entitled to attention at no cost in community health centers and public hospitals run by the government.

For more than ninety years, the Pan American Health Organization/World Health Organization (PAHO/WHO) has maintained a strong presence in the eighteen countries of Latin America and in Puerto Rico. The purpose of PAHO/WHO is "to promote and coordinate the efforts of the countries of the Region of the Americas to combat disease, lengthen life, and promote the physical and mental health of their people" (PAHO 2000). PAHO maintains an office in each of these countries and supports regional training and research centers to improve the health and living conditions of the population of Latin America.

The efforts of PAHO are summarized in the 2000 Annual Report of the Director that states,

> Progress is reflected in steady improvements in
> such national indicators of well-being as life
> expectancy, easy access to safe water supply,
> and immunization coverage, and in reductions
> in health-ill outcomes, particularly the reduc-
> tion of child mortality due to communicable
> diseases.

Through the collaborative efforts of governmental health agencies and PAHO, the main causes of death have shifted from infectious diseases to chronic, non-communicable diseases in most countries.

Because resources are limited, the emphasis of health programs is on preventive care, and these programs cover not only urban areas but rural sectors of countries as well. People living in rural areas are often classified as highly vulnerable or at risk and tend to receive special attention from ministries of health throughout the region. PAHO experts work closely with the health agencies of each country to support the planning, implementation, monitoring, and evaluation of health programs.

Few immigrants from Latin America, then, have poor health. The healthy migrant effect and the epidemiological paradox that were discussed in chapter 1 are clear consequences of having lived in a paternalistic system that promotes preventive health measures. Therefore, practitioners should not be surprised to encounter immigrant Latinos with excellent health. These patients will often have high levels of awareness regarding preventive care.

Latino Definitions of the Causes of Illness

Depending on the level of contact experienced with the health care system, Latinos' explanations of illness may involve a combination of several perspectives. One view of illness is based on the health and disease model that has been discussed. Illness is the absence of health because of an imbalance among the body's humors.

Another commonly found view attributes illness to a supernatural or psychological cause. Illness may also be interpreted as a folk disease.

Supernatural Causes

The causes of some illnesses are found outside the body. The evil eye (*mal de ojo*) is the most common example. Typically, a healthy child whose good looks and health are admired by family, neighbors, and strangers alike develops a persistent fever, general malaise, irritability, and sleepiness. The cause of the child's illness is often attributed to a person with a strong gaze who looked at the child. Many also believe that not having "protection" against the evil eye increases a good-looking child's vulnerability. Parents may use any of a number of artifacts to protect their children from the evil eye, for example, a red-colored thread around a wrist, a cross on a necklace, or garlic cloves in a small pouch hung around the neck.

Psychological Causes

The onset of psychologically induced illnesses results from the person having experienced strong emotional states, such as fright (*susto*) and hysteria (*ataque de nervios*).

The cause of susto is a frightful experience. A woman who is informed that her husband has been seriously injured in an automobile accident may develop restlessness while sleeping, listlessness, anorexia, and disinterest in her personal appearance. Although the woman may later find out that her husband is going to be okay, her symptoms might persist for an indefinite period of time. In some cases the situation may not only persist but may also develop into disinterest in personal hygiene, loss of strength, depression, and introversion.

Ataque de nervios may occur as a consequence of the loss of the love of a boyfriend or girlfriend, of infidelity, or of an impassioned verbal argument. It consists of uncontrolled shaking, profuse perspiration, and sustained and out-of-control screaming that may last for several hours. In addition the person might fall on the floor, may need to be held by others, or may have to be restrained to avoid self-injury. At the end of the episode, although conscious, the patient may lie immobile with both eyes closed. A fluttering of both eyelids is common.

Folk Diseases

In the Latino culture women and children are seen as weaker than men. Consequently, some believe they are more vulnerable to folk diseases. The most common of these conditions are upset stomach (*empacho*) and fallen fontanelle (*mollera caída*). Although both diseases have folk names and meanings, they often have a biological basis and should be considered seriously.

Patients describe the symptoms of empacho as having a sense of fullness, as though having just ingested a large amount of food. The symptoms may persist for several hours or even days. The organic causes of empacho must be explored carefully because they may range from indigestion to appendicitis.

Depressed fontanelle, or mollera caída, is often seen in dehydrated newborns and infants. In these patients the anterior fontanelle is depressed below the contour of the skull as a consequence of the severe loss of fluids due to vomiting, fever, or diarrhea. Poorly educated individuals and people of rural origin believe the cause of the condition to be the palpation of the child's fontanelle during the physical evaluation. Parents who have a low educational level may try home or folk remedies before deciding to take the child to the hospital, thus increasing the mortality rate for newborns and infants.

Latino Health Care Practices

The perceived severity of an illness and the level of education are important factors in a Latino's decision regarding when and who to ask for help. Although educational level strongly influences a Latino's decision to seek health care services, hopelessness due to illnesses with bad prognoses may lead even well-educated Latinos to seek the assistance of folk healers. The traditional healers become a last resort when hopes of reversing a declining health condition diminish.

The believed cause of an illness often determines which type of help someone will seek; in particular, mental illnesses demand special attention. Some Puerto Ricans, for example, believe mental problems are caused by bad spirits and must therefore be dealt with by a person who specializes in spirits. Thus, the preferred provider may be an *espiritista*, a *santero(a)*, or a *curandero(a)* (see pages 62–63 for an explantion).

The most common health-seeking options are self-care, religion, folk medicine, and biomedical care.

Self-Care

Latinos frequently rely on family and friends for advice to treat a condition that they perceive to be of minor severity, such as a sore throat, mild diarrhea, toothache, or a mild skin rash. Self-treatment with home remedies is the method of choice to treat these illnesses, which are expected to disappear in a couple of days. Leftover medication is often used to treat symptoms that appear similar to those for which treatment has been previously prescribed.

Religion

The Catholic religion strongly impacts the health-seeking behaviors of a large number of Catholic Latinos. Seeking the help of God to prevent or cure illness is common among Latinos. This help can be invoked by making promises, visiting shrines, offering medals and candles, and offering prayers. In some cases Latinos use these alternatives exclusively, but in most instances, depending on the perceived severity of the health problem, they may use two or more options simultaneously.

Promises: Making a promise to God is a form of negotiating, asking for improved health in exchange for giving up something that the person enjoys or values highly. An alcoholic father whose baby boy is diagnosed with leukemia might promise God to give up alcohol in exchange for his son's health. A woman whose mother is terminally ill with cancer may prom-

ise God she will never play the lottery again if her
mother's health improves.

While promises are generally offered after a serious diagnosis is made and a bad prognosis is given,
some Latinos also make promises to prevent illness. A
mother might therefore promise God not to give her
child a haircut until the baby is one year old as long as
the child is in good health, or a man might promise
God to wear a purple-colored robe every year on the
day of a given saint to show gratitude to God for his
family's good health.

Visiting Shrines: Latinos visit shrines for two health-
related reasons: to ask God to heal a family member or
to thank God for a favorable health outcome. The visit
to a shrine is usually a family affair in which young
and old share a trip to a faraway shrine to show a
humble attitude before the saint's statue in the shrine.
Real sacrifices may be involved. For example, a family
might decide to walk several kilometers on foot to visit
a shrine. As part of the visit, adults may wear robes
made to be particularly scratchy and uncomfortable in
hopes that the sacrifice will please the saint. Some even
enter the shrine on their bleeding knees to present
themselves before the saint. The fervor with which
some Latinos carry out the visits reflects their faith in
the healing powers of a given saint.

Offering Medals and Lighting Candles: The practice of
making offerings is very common throughout Latin
America. A parent whose child is receiving medical
treatment for a badly fractured leg may offer a medal
to God or to a saint. Upon recovery, the parent and

child take a silver or gold medal in the shape of a leg and pin it to the robe of the saint's statue in their church. They may also light a candle to keep the statue "with light." In some churches, saints' statues that have many candles lighted often indicate the miraculous powers attributed to them. The sight of such a well-illuminated statue stimulates churchgoers to comment on the powers of the given saint. Again, sacrifice is involved; offering a gold medal to a saint represents a financial sacrifice for a parent.

Offering Prayers: For the same reasons that candles and medals are offered, prayers also represent an important health-seeking resource for some Latinos, especially when trying to overcome severe illnesses such as cancer. There are simple and elaborate modalities of prayer. A devoted mother might pray for several hours every day at home or in church. A small or large group of neighbors and friends might pray together every night for nine days. Their prayers are called novenas because they take nine days. The time spent organizing and carrying out the novenas is a clear statement of the willingness of those offering the prayers to make a sacrifice in exchange for the recovery of a dear one.

Offering Masses: Although less frequently mentioned in the literature, offering masses is a very common practice among Catholic Latinos. A family may offer a mass to ask or thank God for a family member's recovery from a diagnosed illness. In this case, a mass also becomes a social event in which friends and neighbors participate.

Folk Medicine

As mentioned earlier, throughout the Spanish colonial period and thereafter, the European humoral theory became closely entwined with the indigenous American Indian herbal medicine practiced throughout most of the Latin American region. Cuba, the Dominican Republic, Puerto Rico, and Haiti were recipients of large numbers of African immigrants brought as slaves. African immigrants enriched the options for managing illnesses in these countries. Thus, folk medicine evolved into a combination of the European humoral theory, the indigenous herbal medicines, and the African view of demons and spirits as the instigators of illness.

The following are the most common folk healing methods used by Latinos. Some are used in combination and others exclusively, depending on the degree of credibility of the provider and on the person's faith in a particular method.

Curanderos. The roots of *curanderismo* are found in Aztec, Spanish, spiritualistic, homeopathic, and scientific practices. It is practiced throughout most of the countries of Latin America and in the U.S. Latino community. As a system of healing, curanderismo considers the patient's health problems as well as his or her cultural and religious beliefs. Curanderos mostly prescribe herb teas and herb baths and perform cleanings, or *limpias*, by passing a broken egg or a batch of herbs tied in a bunch over the person's body.

Curanderos are highly regarded citizens in the community. They establish a personal relationship with the patients, who often confide in and consult with the female or male curandero(a) regarding a wide variety of personal issues. The curanderos generally prefer to work by referral from another patient and may refuse to see a patient they don't like or whom they don't know very well. Curanderos are often referred to as "Maestros."

Sobadores. *Sobadores* are massage therapists who are especially preferred by Latinos of Mexican origin.

Santeros(as) and Espiritistas. Santeros(as) and espiritistas practice *espiritismo* to heal patients. They act as spiritualist mediums to help patients get rid of the spirits. Some Puerto Ricans, for example, believe that spirits located outside the body cause mental illnesses. The origin of Santeria is found among the Africans who came as slaves to the continent of the Americas. It is a popular practice mostly seen in Brazil, Cuba, and Puerto Rico and less throughout the rest of Latin America.

Herbal Healers. Herbal healers operate small community herb pharmacies. They carry a large selection of herbs as well as rosemary water, Florida water, Maravilla water, incense, candles, and religious items. Although these healers fill the prescriptions of espiritistas, it is not uncommon to find herbal healers who prescribe their own remedies. They are very selective with regard to their own clientele.

Biomedical Care

Five compelling symptoms will prompt most Latinos to seek medical care: bleeding, severe pain, persistent high fever, a lump, or the inability to pass stools or urine. Regardless of the reason, Latinos' access to the health care system is strongly influenced by five factors: finances, culture, education, legal status, and geography. Each of the following five vignettes illustrates a lack of access.

Financial Access. Rosa is a third-generation, pregnant Latina of Mexican origin living in San Diego. She works for a company that has offered health insurance. Yet, she has been unable to get coverage because she cannot afford it. Her financial constraints prevent her from seeking health care. Instead, she goes to Tijuana for prenatal care.

Cultural Access. Marta, a high school senior Latina, lives across the street from the hospital where she has health insurance coverage. Instead of requesting an appointment with a primary care professional at the health maintenance organization of which she is a plan member, she opts to use a home remedy suggested by her mother to improve the regularity of her menses. In the Latino culture the mother's role includes caring for her children and solving health problems that may be considered of minor importance by the mother. Thus, culture prevails.

Educational Access. Adan is a twenty-year-old, uneducated legal immigrant from rural Mexico who works as a gardener. His sister made it possible for him to come to the country, get a job, and have health insurance coverage. While working, he cuts his hand. Not knowing what to do, he goes to the neighborhood produce store, buys a bottle of a home remedy imported from Mexico, and applies it to the wound. Three days later he is running a very high temperature. He tells his sister he is feeling very sick, and she takes him to the hospital.

Legal Access. Roberto is a thirty-five-year-old, upper-class plastic surgeon who recently emigrated from Argentina. While preparing to take the medical boards to be certified to practice in the United States, he develops a peptic ulcer. Because he is not yet a legal permanent resident of the U.S., he is not working. Therefore, because he does not have health insurance and does not want to go to a public hospital, he must self-medicate with an over-the-counter medication.

Geographical Access. Jose is a twenty-four-year-old, second-generation, male Latino college student working as a sales representative in a store. When he suffers a severe blow to his arm, he decides not to seek emergency medical attention, although he has health insurance coverage, because the nearest hospital is located very far away from his home and he does not own a car. Instead, he self-medicates by taking an over-the-counter painkiller and applying ice to the swollen arm.

Finally, it must be stated that *Latinos' use of a biomedical provider does not exclude the use of folk medicine providers or other health care options.* The perceived warmth and the caring attitude of the provider, described as simpatía or personalismo, often determines the preference of the patient and the patient's family to visit a clinician a second time. In other words, the degree of rapport established during the first interaction largely determines the patient's satisfaction with the health care provider.

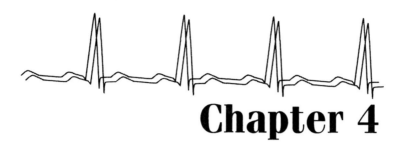

Chapter 4

Communicating Effectively with the Latino Patient

Delivering health messages to Latinos can be a challenging undertaking because of the diversity of the group. "Creative and innovative communication materials and strategies are needed" (Ramirez and Baraona 1997). Three issues are important for a provider who is attempting to give health information to a Latino patient during the clinical encounter. First, it is useful to have a clear picture of the risk factors that have an impact on Latinos' health and to understand how acculturation can have deleterious effects on Latinos' health (Sabogal et al. 1996). Second, it is essential to understand how cultural issues may act as protective factors and how health care practitioners may use preventive messages effectively (Baezconde-Garbanati et al. 1999; Perez-Stable et al. 1998). Third, delivering information through a "sharing experience'" may enhance the impact of the messages.

Risk Factors and Acculturation

The most important risk factors among Latinos are alcohol and tobacco use, nutritional habits, and lack of exercise. In a snapshot, this is the situation:

Alcohol and Tobacco

⇒ Men drink more heavily after immigrating.

⇒ Latino males smoke less as they become acculturated.

⇒ With each generation beyond immigration, women of Mexican origin living in the United States are drinking and smoking more.

⇒ Although only 17 percent of Latinas smoke, 27.2 percent of Latina high school students report that they are smokers.

⇒ Mexican women drink more than Puerto Rican and Cuban American women.

⇒ Sixty-two percent of third-generation and 49 percent of second-generation Mexican American women drink, compared with only 25 percent of immigrant Mexican women.

(Casas et al. 1998; Marin and Posner 1995; Black and Markides 1993; Gilbert 1991; Cervantes et al.

1991; Marin et al. 1990; Johnson and Delgado 1989; Ramirez and McAlister 1988.)

Nutritional Habits and Lack of Exercise

⇒ There is no typical Latino diet. However, many Latinos' diets have lower fat and higher fiber content than the diets of non-Latino whites.

⇒ Less-acculturated Latinos are more likely to eat fruits, rice, beans, meat, and fried foods and to drink whole milk more often than more acculturated Latinos are.

⇒ As they become more acculturated, Latinos' diets become a key factor in the prevalence of obesity, diabetes, and hypertension.
(Alcalay et al. 1999; Otero-Sabogal et al. 1995; Alcalay et al. 1992.)

Conveying Health Messages Successfully

Understanding and addressing cultural values may act as a bridge toward helping the provider communicate health information effectively (Perez-Stable et al. 1998; Ramirez and Baraona 1997; Moreno et al. 1997; Balcazar et al. 1995; Alcalay et al. 1993). Four cultural values are critical in reaching Latinos with educational health messages: familism, friends, faith, and fatalism. The first two can help initiate behavioral change and the latter two may help guide and maintain the process of change.

Familism

In contrast with the individualistic nature of the American mainstream culture, Latinos, as discussed in chapter 1, view their world from a family perspective; therefore, suggesting that a patient stop smoking for the purpose of improving personal health is not generally an effective way of communicating the message. Rather, appealing to the well-being of the family should be a major component of the message to a patient. The following ten family-related reasons are more likely to motivate a smoker to change his or her behavior.

1. To spare suffering to the family
2. To save money for a family vacation
3. To have good breath and avoid being rejected by one's spouse
4. To protect family members from secondhand smoke
5. To have the pleasure of knowing and playing with grandchildren in the future
6. To set a good example for children
7. To gain more respect from family members
8. To be a responsible provider for the family
9. To avoid having arguments with parents
10. To gain attention from family members

Friends

The Latino culture attaches great value to the larger collective, one's friends as well as one's family. A Latino person's behavior is often guided by the attitudes and advice of his or her friends. For example, a Latino or

Latina is generally dependent on friends and relatives and is often more concerned about trust, empathy, and the welfare of the group than mainstream U.S. Americans are. The *social network has a high priority; being competitive and achievement-oriented is less important.* Thus, suggesting that a Latino patient set the personal goal to stop drinking may not produce positive results. In contrast, alluding to issues related to friends may make a greater impact on the patient, helping to initiate behavioral change. A recommendation to start attending Alcoholics Anonymous meetings using the following justifications can be useful:

1. To be able to help friends who have the same problem
2. To show friends the force of personal willpower
3. To be able to influence friends
4. To understand friends
5. To be accepted by friends
6. To avoid being rejected by the social group
7. To meet new friends

Faith

Religious faith and faith in the provider are two powerful resources that can be called upon when delivering a health message. Many Latinos believe most of their problems will be solved because they have faith in God. Thus, they may believe that hypertension will be controlled because of all the prayers offered to God, the Virgin Mary, or to a favorite saint. Or they may be confident that their health will improve because of their steadfast trust in the abilities of their health provider.

Faith in a provider is a development of either many years of consulting with that person or it is a consequence of a situation in which the provider is believed to have saved a patient's life. In either case such a patient may perceive health advice as highly credible or may follow through with advice if the provider alludes to the patient's faith in God. Some examples will be helpful.

1. An overweight Mexican woman who begins an exercise and diet program because the Virgin of Guadalupe is looking after her
2. A retired elderly man who carefully monitors his blood pressure because the nurse is always very accurate in her advice
3. A Puerto Rican man who joins a smoking cessation program because God sent him to the social worker
4. A teenager's mother who has faith in the provider's ability to get her son off drugs

Fatalism

Of these four Latino values, fatalism is the one that may work against health care providers, the one they may have to work hard to bypass or overcome. Succeeding in the face of fatalistic arguments is difficult because most Latinos avoid confrontations. The best approach is to speak about alternatives to broaden the patient's perspective instead of trying to talk the patient out of the belief that an event is predetermined and unalterable. When a patient unites faith and fatalism, the challenge is even greater because of the belief that God is determining his or her fate, and therefore there is nothing to be done. Here are some examples of alternatives that may help.

1. Even though the outcome may be predetermined, it won't hurt the patient to try....
2. A patient may want to make sure that an event is really unalterable.
3. God may have a change of mind in view of the patient's efforts to improve his or her health.
4. A saint may be impressed with the patient's faith and acceptance and may decide to help reverse the condition.
5. There may be other missions in life that the person may still have to accomplish and pulling through this illness may be one.
6. God may be trying to test the patient's faith.

The provider's understanding of Latino values and the ability to make those values work in the patient's favor can be useful in stirring the pot and capturing a Latino patient's interest. The patient can then be motivated to take action to improve and maintain a healthy lifestyle.

Sharing: A Key Element in Reaching Latinos

Sharing is at the core of Latino collectivism. People plan weekends with the family to be together and to share. Men drink with friends. Women talk to other women in the community to share information. Teenage girls smoke with their friends because they want to share. Thus, it makes sense that giving preventive messages to a patient may be most effective when it becomes a sharing experience. The highly respected provider shares knowledge with the patient and shows concern. The patient shares personal health problems. Together, provider and patient identify feasible ways that can help achieve behavioral change that will help protect the patient's health.

How does a provider accomplish a "sharing experience"? It depends on the clinician's personal style. In essence, sharing involves being able to listen to the patient, create a harmonious conversation, establish a personal relationship, give advice using as many examples as possible, and always encourage the patient to ask questions. The examples are used to illustrate points and may be taken from personal or family experience. The only precondition to the degree of sharing is the length of time the provider has known the patient and the degree of personal trust perceived from the patient. If the patient is new, it is always better to listen more and suggest less. Sharing is at its best when a strong patient-provider relationship has been established and the patient has developed trust in the provider.

Motivating the Latino Patient to Adopt Healthy Habits

Three factors may contribute to motivating a Latino patient to adopt a healthier lifestyle: knowing the health education priorities of Latinos, understanding what type of information is appealing to Latinos, and individualizing the information to the extent that the patient perceives it as a customized message that touches him or her personally.

Health Education Priorities

The National Coalition of Hispanic Health and Human Services Organizations proposed seven areas as the health promotion needs of Latino communities (Delgado 1998):

1. Supporting positive prenatal care practices among Latinas
2. Linking prenatal care services to well-baby care with special attention to generational differences
3. Providing information about childhood immunization programs to parents
4. Providing parents with information on adequate access to and management of chronic childhood conditions, particularly asthma and lead exposure
5. Delivering effective accident and injury prevention and traffic safety programs
6. Developing peer and family-focused programs to support adolescents in positive life choices regarding family planning, substance abuse (use of tobacco, alcohol, and inhalants), violence, and suicide prevention
7. Developing health promotion programs for adults that support the management of chronic and disabling conditions, particularly diabetes, heart disease, cancer, HIV/AIDS, liver disease, and conditions arising from environmental hazards

Providers and educators should also be aware of the fact that prior to immigrating to the United States, Latinos may have been recipients of health messages that addressed health issues differently. In the U.S., health is seen as an individual responsibility, but in most Latin American countries public health is framed as a collective responsibility of the state, providers, and family members. In these countries, health messages often *strongly suggest specific behavioral changes*. In contrast, upon immigrating to the U.S., patients are presented with messages that *suggest options* to improve health.

Information that Is Appealing to Latinos

The most important considerations in making information appealing to Latinos are effectiveness, sensitivity, channel, and a positive approach. First, the most effective way to deliver health-related information to Latinos is to use simple language, short sentences, many illustrations and examples, and testimonials (Alcalay et al. 1992). For example, twelve tablespoons of grease are more readily visualized than 200 grams of fat. By the same token, four ounces of beef are better described as a piece of meat the size of a pack of cards. Second, information should reflect sensitivity to the degree to which the patient has acculturated and to the generation of the patient (Bell and Alcalay 1997; Gilbert 1991). Although a second-generation Latina may visualize herself exercising in a gym, an immigrant from Central America may best relate to exercise when the provider suggests that she walk an extra block to the bus stop. Third, use the channel preferred by Latinos, who give higher credibility to information received from physicians, family, and friends (Marin 1996).

Finally, health messages are most attractive when the focus is health and not disease or its consequences. The positive approach is less intimidating and more inviting.

Individualized and Personalized Information

The lifestyles of many Latinos are plagued with difficulties related to family commitments, time management, and acculturative stress. Therefore, certain health promotion suggestions may sound unreasonable. To recommend an exercise regime when a person is hectically trying to cope with a tight, two-job work schedule while facing the stress of learning a new language and adjusting to life in a new country would nearly guarantee that the health message would be ignored.

Latinos often accept health advice willingly, but they most appreciate customized information. For example, instead of giving a detailed explanation of the benefits of exercise, it works best to ask the patient about past attempts to engage in exercise programs. Knowing that the practitioner is not delivering a packaged message but rather personal advice makes a patient feel important and cared for.

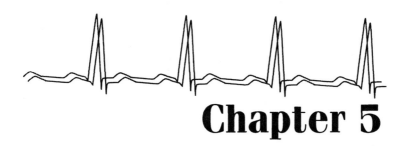

Chapter 5

Achieving Cultural Competence with the Latino Patient

The critical point of encounter between health care organizations and multicultural populations is the clinical setting. Thus, providers are key actors in the delivery of care that responds to the needs of culturally diverse patients (Ailinger and Dear 1997; Humphry et al. 1997). While the demand for minority physicians continues to increase (Saha et al. 2000), so does the need to equip clinicians with cultural competency tools to help enhance communication with their culturally diverse patients.

Cultural Competence

To understand Latino culture, a more basic understanding of the meaning of *culture* is critical (National Alli-
ance for Hispanic Health 2001). Culture is "learned,
shared, and transmitted values, beliefs, norms, and
lifeways of a designated group which are generally
transmitted intergenerationally and influence one's
thinking and action modes" (Leininger 1995). Central
to the process of attaining cultural competence is personal experience regarding culture, both yours and the
patient's. It is reasonable to assume that cultural competence is not something that occurs instinctually. It
must be learned, and the first step in that process is to
define the concept.

At the end of 2000, after culminating a process of
consultation, the Office of Minority Health released
the standards for culturally and linguistically appropriate services in health care. These standards define
cultural and linguistic competence and address the
nationwide concerns of health care organizations that
provide services to the diverse U.S. population.

"Cultural and linguistic competence suggests an
ability by health care providers and health care organizations to understand and respond effectively to the
cultural and linguistic needs brought by patients to the
health care encounter" (Office of Minority Health
2000). This definition is broad in its perspective and
attempts to incorporate many of the issues raised by
academic, professional, and health care organizations.
For example, the American Medical Association de-

fines culturally competent physicians as follows: "Culturally competent physicians are able to provide patient-centered care by adjusting their attitudes and behaviors to account for the impact of emotional, cultural, social, and psychological issues on the main biomedical ailment" (1999). In an article published in the *American Journal of Nursing*, the authors posit,

> If the nursing profession is to address the needs of all patients, nurses must understand that cultural competence does not mean substituting one's own cultural identity with another (which suggests that cultural traits can be easily shed), ignoring the variability within cultural groups, or even knowing everything about the cultures being served. Instead, a respect for difference, an eagerness to learn, and a willingness to accept that there are many ways of viewing the world will distinguish nurses who integrate cultural competence into their daily practice from those who merely understand it. (Gonzalez et al. 2000)

From a social worker's perspective, cultural competency is defined as

> the set of knowledge and skills that a social worker must develop in order to be effective with multicultural clients. The culturally competent person has the task of bringing together elements from his or her culture of origin and the dominant culture to accomplish bicultural integration and competency. (Lum 1999)

The most concise definition of cultural competence comes from Mikel Hogan-Garcia: "the ability to interact effectively with diverse people" (1999).

Steps toward Achieving Cultural Competence

Attaining cultural competence encompasses a personal process that leads to acquiring skills through self-awareness, cultural knowledge of others, self-reflection, and practice. Various models of cultural competence exist (Lum 1999; Hogan-Garcia 1999; Campinha-Bacote 1994; Bennett 1993; Cross et al. 1989), but most authors agree on at least four closely linked and sequential steps: cultural awareness, cultural knowledge, cultural skills, and inductive learning.

1. *Cultural Awareness:* Developing cultural awareness involves a personal commitment to becoming aware of one's own culture and that of the Latino patient. The process of examining and confronting personal biases or assumptions regarding Latinos often leads to the development of cultural sensitivity.

2. *Cultural Knowledge:* Having access to and studying information about the health status of Latinos and their cultural values is the second step, an invaluable element in helping the practitioner understand and explain issues that arise during the clinical encounter.

3. *Cultural Skills:* Developing cultural skills is a consequence of having reflected about cultural awareness and of gaining knowledge about the Latino culture. The most important element here, though,

is *practicing* what has been learned. Part II of this book offers the first segment of this skill building: vignettes that illustrate cultural skills as applied in the health care encounter.

4. *Inductive Learning:* The sensitive provider's frequent clinical interaction with Latino patients reinforces his or her skill development and, if mindfully applied to the principles of cultural competence, leads to a greater understanding of the culture.

Latino Cultural Competence Self-Assessment Tool

Attaining effective communication with a Latino patient can lead to a satisfactory clinical encounter for patient and provider. Good communication can impact the quality of health services and may lead to achieving positive health outcomes for the patient. Undoubtedly, provider satisfaction is also important, especially when the health care system faces so many challenges. Where should a clinician start the journey toward cultural competence?

A suggested first step is to carry out an exploratory self-assessment of one's cultural competency with Latino patients. To my knowledge, a tool of this kind does not exist; the assessment of cultural competence is still an emerging issue. Three more general assessment tools, however, have promising applicability to the Latino culture. Doman Lum's comprehensive "Social Work Cultural Competencies Self-Assessment" includes 44 close-ended questions that evaluate the social work student's *level* of cultural competency on a scale of 1–4 (1999). Miguel Tirado's "Provider's Self-Assessment Tool" emerged from research with Latino and Chinese patients and physicians. It is intended for use with physicians and other health care providers working in a managed care system. Its 18 close-ended questions are intended to determine the *degree* to which providers could benefit from further training or experience in providing culturally competent health care (Tirado 1996). Elena Cohen and Tawara Goode's "Cultural Competence Self-Test" consists of a checklist for primary health care services personnel and was designed to help physicians in identifying *areas* in which they might improve the quality of their services to multicultural populations (Cohen and Goode 1999).

In the next section I present a Latino cultural competency assessment tool that draws elements from the three tools mentioned above. It is a step toward the development of a full-fledged self-assessment tool to measure cultural competency specifically with Latino patients. This preliminary instrument consists of a set of twenty statements. The first ten *true* or *false* items evaluate the provider's *knowledge* of the Latino culture in the clinical environment. The last ten items ask the provider to choose between three options: "often," "sometimes," and "rarely" and evaluate the provider's *skills* in communicating with Latino patients. I hope that the responses may help the provider establish his or her cultural competence level with Latino patients. The answers to the questions are found on page 87.

Cultural Competence with Latino Patients

Knowledge

1. The three highest mortality rates among Latinos are diseases of the heart, cancer, and accidents.

      True   False

2. The three major health problems of Latinos are diabetes, tuberculosis, and HIV infection.

      True   False

3. The "healthy migrant effect" attempts to explain the higher mortality rates of immigrants from Latin America.

      True   False

4. Diet is a health risk factor only for Latinas.

      True   False

5. With increased acculturation, Latinas drink more heavily but smoke fewer cigarettes.

      True   False

6. Visiting shrines and offering masses are important health practices of some Latinos.

      True   False

7. Mollera caída is a folk disease but not a true health condition.

      True   False

8. A patient with empacho may have acute appendicitis.

      True   False

9. Some Puerto Ricans believe mental diseases are associated with spirits.

True   False

10. Persons of Mexican origin may have high regard for a curandero's or sobadore's healing abilities.

True   False

Personal Interaction Skills

11. Making eye contact while shaking hands is at the top of my list when greeting a Latino patient.

Often   Sometimes   Rarely

12. I avoid asking the patient direct questions when inquiring about the cause for consultation.

Often   Sometimes   Rarely

13. I ask the patient if he or she prefers to take the medication in tablet, capsule, or liquid form.

Often   Sometimes   Rarely

14. I try to encourage the patient's relatives to stay in the office during the consultation.

Often   Sometimes   Rarely

15. When seeking consent for a special procedure, I include the patient's family.

Often   Sometimes   Rarely

16. I try to determine if an elderly Latino patient is to be informed of the diagnosis before I disclose it.

Often   Sometimes   Rarely

17. I walk the patient to the door at the end of the consultation.

   Often   Sometimes   Rarely

18. When giving a rectal examination to a male Latino, I try to consider the patient's cultural issues.

   Often   Sometimes   Rarely

19. I address patients with titles such as "Mr.," "Mrs.," or "Miss."

   Often   Sometimes   Rarely

20. I include the patient's family when I give advice to the patient.

   Often   Sometimes   Rarely

Answers to Self-Assessment Questions

   1. True
   2. True
   3. False
   4. False
   5. False
   6. True
   7. False
   8. True
   9. True
   10. True

Questions 11–20: Although there are no correct answers, the "often" response reflects highly desirable interactive skills with Latino patients.

The intersection between the cultural values of the Latino population and the definition of cultural competence suggested by the Office of Minority Health presents a challenging picture of the clinical encounter.

First, it would be difficult for a practitioner to respond to a Latino patient's cultural needs with only basic knowledge of Latino cultural values, even assuming that linguistic resources were readily available. For example, a clinician who understands that familism is a central cultural value for Latinos might not be able to understand and respond effectively to a patient without knowing that he or she came to this country fleeing a civil war.

Second, an arsenal of tools is needed to develop cultural competence, and such skills must be learned through specific training in Latino cultural competence rather than through generic cultural competence training. This approach should render positive results. As David Hayes-Bautista et al. stated,

> While it is vitally important to increase the number of Latino physicians, it is equally important to train non-Latino physicians in culturally effective ways to provide medical care. Latino patients can present a number of paradoxes to physicians who are not trained to manage them. Yet, culturally prepared physicians report a high degree of mutual bloom. And continuing medical education can provide cultural effectiveness education for providers already in practice. (1999)

In conclusion, developing cultural competence with Latino patients requires a close look at the cultural and personal characteristics that the patient brings to the encounter. The cultural traits may be known, but the unique personal issues, closely linked to culture but specific of each individual's life experience, must also be identified. The Latino Culturally Competent Care Model presented in the second part of this book addresses these issues. The model suggests a practical approach to use during each stage of the clinical encounter with a Latino patient. The intention of the first part of this book has been to act as a catalyst to facilitate the journey of providers by raising cultural *awareness* and providing cultural *knowledge* that may guide providers as they increase their sensitivity toward Latino patients. The second part of the book presents a practice-oriented perspective to describe the steps that are most appropriate to develop the *skills* needed to interact effectively with a Latino patient.

Dos and Don'ts with Latino Patients

Dos

⇒ Do expect the patient to have a definition of health that reflects a combination of cultures.

⇒ Do understand that God and the family lie at the center of the patient's life.

Don'ts

⇒ Don't smile when a patient is discussing health beliefs. It may be perceived as lack of respect.

⇒ Don't ask the patient to explain the reasons that support his/her health beliefs. The patient may interpret that the provider has doubts regarding the cultural basis of the beliefs.

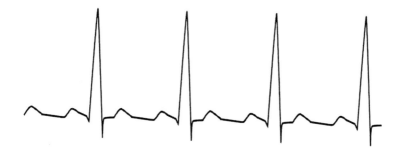

Part II

A Culturally Competent Care Model for Latinos

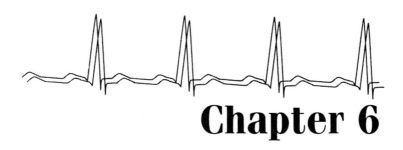

Chapter 6

GREET:
Characterizing
Your Latino Patient

It is useful to characterize a Latino patient for two reasons. First, such information gathering helps you gain
insight into the patient's background while increasing
opportunities to know the personal and cultural bag-
gage that the patient brings to the encounter. Knowing a patient's personal and cultural issues helps the
provider understand what led the patient to seek health
care.

Second, Latinos welcome providers' interest in
gathering information and perceive it as a sign of personal attention that increases the patient's perception
of being respected. This chapter will help you to es-

tablish the right tone in an initial meeting and to identify cultural issues that have implications for the
patient's health.

The Clinical Encounter

The groundwork for the patient-provider relationship
is laid from the moment the patient walks into the
provider's office. When a non-Latino provider meets a
Latino patient in the clinical setting, both face the
challenges of a cross-cultural interaction. For the provider, having cultural skills is essential in order to attain a satisfactory provider-patient encounter. The
patient, on the other hand, may not have enough
knowledge of the language and may also lack familiarity with the local culture.

Although you may be used to a diverse clientele,
this intercultural encounter may be a first experience
for the Latino patient. Situations that present language
and cultural barriers can be uncomfortable for the patient who generally prefers environments with familiar faces and a common culture. A Latino patient who
seeks help from a provider often has a sense of antici-
pation regarding what the culture of the provider will
be. Knowing that almost invariably the provider will
not be a Latino or Latina adds pressure to this first
encounter because if the patient is a first-generation
Latino, he or she may anticipate difficulty in establishing adequate communication. Latino patients often lament their inability to speak English and fear that
it may lead to a provider perceiving them as socially,

educationally, or financially disadvantaged. Being able to "have dignity" is high on Latinos' priority list of factors that surround social interaction, and fear of being perceived as poor or disadvantaged can erode their sense of dignity. Thus, your sensitivity to the extra effort the Latino patient has made to seek help despite language and cultural barriers can help create a welcoming atmosphere in the office.

Often the patient enters the office with hesitation, anxiety, and sometimes, even fear. Hesitation arises from having chosen the option of seeking help from a mainstream provider. Anxiety comes from anticipating the difficulties in communication that are bound to happen. Fear of the unknown and fear of the implications of a serious health problem are also powerful emotions that the Latino patient may be experiencing when he or she walks into the clinic or office.

The greeting is the first contact you have with a patient. It can, therefore, be the crucial factor that determines the success or failure of the patient-provider relationship.

Regardless of your personal communication style, there are a number of factors that should be considered paramount when greeting a Latino patient: eye contact, facial expression, gestures, touch, voice intonation, and the use of titles. The initial questions you ask must also be carefully considered. A provider who understands the importance of these key initial elements of the encounter will be prepared to effectively develop rapport with a Latino patient and will communicate respect.

Eye Contact

Making eye contact with Latino patients is critical. Yet you will want to be careful because gender differences of both patient and provider influence what appropriate eye contact is. For example, a male or female provider should make eye contact briefly with a patient of the opposite sex. A clinician who maintains a sustained gaze at a patient may send the message that he or she is personally attracted to the patient.

In contrast, with a patient of the same sex, eye contact may be more prolonged, but only after the patient is seated. A steady gaze after the patient is settled suggests that the provider is focusing attention exclusively on the patient rather than on filling out forms.

Eye contact is also important when a patient, regardless of gender, is disclosing personal information regarding habits and practices or is explaining the symptoms of an illness. Unhappy Latino patients leaving a provider's office often comment, "The doctor didn't even look at me." Thus, even when using a medical interpreter or when communicating through a relative acting as a translator, eye contact with the patient is essential.

Facial Expression

Your facial expression has the power to convey respect and warmth to a Latino patient. Offering a smile may make a patient feel at ease. However, make an effort to abstain from smiling immediately after the patient has spoken because it may be interpreted as a condescending reaction to the patient's verbal communication.

An unexaggerated, friendly smile combined with brief eye contact can make a Latino patient feel welcome in your office. In contrast, a stern face can create stress by leading the patient to think that you are not happy about the language barrier, the patient's illness, or the patient's culture or ethnicity.

Gestures

Latinos talk with their arms and hands. Gestures are as important as words for Latinos when they communicate.

A provider who stands up to greet a patient is perceived to be showing respect. Greeting a patient while gesturing toward a chair may convey a welcoming message, and not doing so may provoke uncomfortable feelings of rejection. When Latinos receive visitors in their homes, they make special efforts to ask guests to sit down in their living room. They expect similar treatment when visiting a provider's office; being asked to sit down by the provider expresses an inviting and warm message.

Touch

Latinos are used to touching and being touched. They use their hands and arms for physical communication, even with strangers.

A provider who stands up and greets a male or female patient with a handshake while simultaneously placing the left hand on the patient's right hand or arm creates a strong connection with the patient. In most cases a firm and brief handshake is sufficient. This too is perceived as a sign of respect by the patient. Either gesture helps ensure that you will be perceived as simpático, or as being empathetic and people-oriented.

Voice Intonation

The tone with which you speak is critical, especially for Latinos who do not speak the same language as the provider. A provider who speaks in a loud voice may be perceived as ill-tempered, impolite, or upset about having a Latino in the office. On the other hand, a provider with a very soft voice may be perceived as lacking in personality. In the patient's mind, the tone of your voice may connote acceptance or rejection of the patient's ethnicity. This is especially important when using interpreters. In sum, Latino patients appreciate providers who greet them with a warm, friendly, and moderate tone of voice.

Titles

Titles are closely related to the issue of respect. When addressing a Latino patient, a provider (regardless of his or her own age) should always use the title *Señor* (Mr.), *Señora* (Mrs.), or *Señorita* (Miss) preceding either the patient's first or last name. The use of titles is most important to women and older people. Latinos expect to be addressed by their last name in the United States although in Latin America providers frequently address patients by their first names to establish familiarity.

The use of the correct title for a Latina can be a sensitive issue and should be considered carefully. The title "Señorita" strongly implies that the woman is single and a virgin and is therefore a decent and reputable person. The title "Señora" suggests that the woman is married and/or has children and also has good moral reputation.

For example, addressing a single woman as "Mrs." may be potentially disrespectful because it implies that she is an unmarried, yet sexually active woman. Although the reality may be different, in the Latin American tradition a decent woman is expected to remain a virgin until her wedding day. Younger generations of Latinas may not care much about the distinction, but it could nevertheless create discomfort for some. On the other hand, young Latino males are often addressed by first name and without a title.

First Questions

What is the best way to initiate communication while greeting a patient? Asking a simple question such as "How are you?" or "How is the family?" may trigger a long answer because Latinos enjoy talking about their feelings and their families. To elicit the reasons for this visit, it may work best to ask a direct question: "What are your concerns about your health?" Although you may need to use additional probes to obtain more information, the patient will be heading in the right direction. When patients perceive interest on the part of the provider, they may engage in a long conversation to explain how they feel and what their family's health status is. Therefore, it may be useful to ask a more direct question that, while showing genuine interest, may produce more direct answers. There is a fine balance between asking open and direct questions and showing concern. Patients interpret direct questions as a desire to end the visit. Guiding a patient is a matter of courteously interrupting whenever the patient begins to roam toward other subjects.

The next question you might ask is: "What brings you here today?" Normally, a mainstream patient will then focus on the exact problem that triggered the visit. However, it is unlikely that a Latino patient will respond to the question with an immediate, straightforward answer. These are some possible answers a Latino patient might give:

Male teenager:	My parents don't know I'm here.
Male adult:	Well, I'm here at my wife's insistence. I really feel fine.
Elderly male:	My daughter said I should come.
Female teenager:	My mother would kill me if she knew I came to see you.
Female adult:	I need to stay healthy for my children.
Elderly female:	My children think that I should get a checkup.

Although each answer is different, each response reveals the critical importance of family to the Latino patient—and none of them are direct responses to the provider's question. In fact, Latinos expect an ice-breaker question and see it as a good sign on the part of the provider. Patients may later report to family members that the provider was truly caring because

he or she did not "cut to the chase." There is a draw-
back, however.

Time is of prime importance in the current health
care setting; yet, Latino patients often roam while describing their ailments instead of quickly focusing on
what prompted their visit. Being relaxed about time is
a Latino cultural trait. Immediately asking a patient
the reason for the visit is not the best approach for
eliciting information. In the Latino culture such a direct, to-the-point question is often considered improper and may suggest a lack of personal interest on
the part of the provider or a desire to conclude the
appointment rapidly. The patient will resent such behavior and, although it may not be evident to you,
any further attempts at connecting with the patient
are likely to prove unsuccessful. The patient will carry
on until the end of the appointment because seeking
harmonious relations is another Latino cultural value.
However, the patient will most likely leave the office
disappointed, will not comply with suggested treatment, and will seek a new provider.

There is one strategy that seldom fails when a patient engages in discussing matters that appear to be
unrelated to the visit. It combines body language and
spoken language. Putting one hand on the patient's
hand and asking, "What problem bothers you the most
today?" can work wonders. This approach conveys your
personal interest in helping solve the pressing problem. The question usually triggers the long-awaited
answer that elucidates the patient's precise reason for
seeking the consultation.

In order to create a culturally appropriate encounter, you might also mention that later in the visit there will be questions regarding the patient's family. In this way the patient will know that there will be an opportunity to briefly talk about the family. Helping the patient focus on the reason for the visit requires mastering the art of using a set of consecutive questions that dynamically guide the conversation while conveying respect toward the patient and his or her cultural values.

Once the door is opened, you may be able to proceed with any number of direct questions. At this point taking control of the time and selecting questions carefully are critical because of the extended initial segment of the appointment.

GREET: Five Steps to Characterize Your Latino Patient

The GREET approach is a five-item analytical tool that will help you identify cultural issues that have implications for the patient's health. The GREET approach will help you skillfully guide the conversation and obtain critical information. This approach will not only save time but it will also create rapport. The GREET acronym stands for

G = Generation
R = Reason for immigrating to the U.S.
E = Extended or nuclear family
E = Ethnic behavior
T = Time living in the U.S.

Generation

As discussed in chapter 3, determining whether the patient is an immigrant or a second-, third-, or fourth-generation Latino is critical to an overall understanding of the patient. Patients are often very eager to volunteer this information because they are proud to talk about their family's success in moving and adjusting to the country.

Immigrants may describe their struggles and express their hopes regarding the future of their children. Second-generation Latinos often share experiences regarding their parents' efforts to succeed in a new environment. Third- and fourth-generation Latinos are usually mainstream.

As also discussed in chapter 3, critical health implications are associated with each generation. Acculturative stress, lack of job opportunities, and lower access to health care are among the problems recent immigrants face. Second-generation Latinos often feel torn between the health beliefs of their parents and those of the local culture. Third- and fourth-generation Latinos usually share the health beliefs of mainstream America.

Reason for Immigrating to the United States

If the patient is an immigrant, it is useful to briefly explore his or her reason(s) for immigrating. This information may increase your understanding of the social, economic, and political pressures that underlie the patient's physical and mental health status. For example, persons who have fled armed conflicts may have post-traumatic stress syndrome, and persons who come from urban or rural environments may be used to totally different lifestyles (Plante et al. 1995; Hondagneu-Sotelo 1994; Leslie 1993; Salgado de Snyder et al. 1990).

It is best to avoid inquiring about immigration status, however. Even if a patient voluntarily reports having legal immigration documentation, the chance that the patient may have undocumented friends or relatives is high. Discussing immigration issues may create anxiety and hamper possibilities of building a trustful relationship.

Extended or Nuclear Family

Knowing whether the Latino patient lives close to the extended or nuclear family provides valuable information because such family members constitute the social support network (see chapter 2). In Latin America it is customary for extended families to live in the same neighborhoods. Upon moving to the United States, Latinos usually try to maintain the tradition of settling in cities or neighborhoods where family members live.

Recent immigrants are often dependent on their families for housing and basic needs, including health care. Second generation persons, on the other hand, usually rely on parents or other family members to help take care of young children while they are working. Family members often serve as counselors and advisers regarding health matters. Third-generation Latinos may remain emotionally attached to the family even though they might be more geographically distant from relatives due to availability of job opportunities. They tend, however, to be less dependent on the family for health matters.

A patient who does not have a spouse, close relative, or extended family living nearby may have a number of unmet emotional and health needs.

Ethnic Behavior

Investigation of the patient's preferences with respect to food, music, holidays, and recreational activities is important. People of Mexican and Central American origin, for example, may eat more highly spiced, carbohydrate-based meals, and natives of South America usually eat more red meat and vegetables and less spice. Such dietary habits may help guide your understanding of the clinical manifestations of the health problem.

Latinos, both male and female, who like music may be avid partygoers and may consume alcohol and/or tobacco in larger amounts than those less inclined to party. Celebrating both American and other countries' holidays also increases opportunities for greater alcohol use for both genders and may have important health implications.

Time Living in the United States

The longer the patient has lived in the United States, the higher his or her degree of acculturation is likely to be. As mentioned in chapter 1, with higher acculturation levels, lifestyles and health behaviors become more like those of mainstream Americans. Therefore, time living in the U.S. is a good indication of the patient's lifestyle and health habits. In some Latino households, the eating habits of the extended family may help illustrate the point: the grandparents' preference may be tortillas, rice, and beans; the grandchildren may dislike that diet and prefer hamburgers; and the adult parents may like both diets.

In sum, the GREET approach can help you understand the cultural background of a Latino patient, establish rapport, and provide an effective response to the patient's needs. This approach can also contribute to making the encounter a more gratifying experience for both you and the patient. By using the GREET approach, you will be better able to respond effectively to the patient's needs.

GREET in Practice

Practicing the GREET approach requires that the practitioner ask a few open-ended questions, listen carefully, and observe the patient with interest and sensitivity toward his or her culture.

The following two vignettes describe the initial encounters between two non-Latino providers and their Latino patients. The vignettes depict communication situations that illustrate cultural issues in the clinical setting. A discussion of the encounter follows each vignette.

Patient 1: Josefina Rivas

Mrs. Rivas is an eighty-year-old woman of Mexican origin who is brought to the physician's office by her teenage granddaughter. She asks her granddaughter to wait for her outside.

Dr. Chang: Good morning, Señora Rivas. How are you feeling this morning? (Dr. Chang smiles and briefly holds Mrs. Rivas' hand.)

Mrs. Rivas: Oh, I'm feeling very sad and lonely. I don't even listen to my music anymore.

Dr. Chang: How is your appetite?

Mrs. Rivas: I don't eat much these days. I only eat because my daughter says I have to, but I don't feel like eating my enchiladas like I used to when I was young. I was very pretty when I was young, you know. That's what my husband used to say. When we came here from Mexico in 1940, I was twenty and my husband was thirty. We were poor, but we were so happy. I miss him so much, God took him two years ago. I had to move in with my daughter and her family. They have an extra bedroom because my oldest grandson got married and moved next door. But she's always so busy with the other children.

Dr. Chang: What health problem brings you to
               my office today? (Dr. Chang makes
               eye contact as he asks the question.)

Mrs. Rivas: I want to go to Mexico for Christ-
               mas, but I have this pain in my legs. I
               don't have good circulation; my
               daughter says I have sugar in my
               blood. I also have a lot of itchiness
               in my private parts.

Using the GREET Approach

Dr. Chang listened and observed Mrs. Rivas as she spoke. He collected valuable information that gave him important clues to understanding the factors affecting Mrs. Rivas' health.

Generation. Mrs. Rivas is an elderly Mexican woman who immigrated to the U.S. in 1940.

Reason. Mrs. Rivas and her husband probably immigrated for economic reasons.

Extended or nuclear family. Mrs. Rivas is a widow and lives with her daughter and her family. She misses her spouse and depends on her daughter.

Ethnic behavior. She is used to eating her Mexican food and may not be following a special diet.

Time living in the U.S. She has lived in the U.S. at least sixty years. Yet, she is very attached to the Mexican culture.

Key Points

⇒ Mrs. Rivas' request that her granddaughter wait for
    her outside indicated to Dr. Chang that she needed

privacy to talk about a personal matter or believed she needed the doctor to examine her in private.

⇒ Dr. Chang used the first two questions as ice-breakers. Yet, they triggered answers that revealed the patient's emotional state. Instead of describing how she is feeling physically, Mrs. Rivas shares that she is lonely and unhappy.

⇒ The third question encourages Mrs. Rivas to focus on and talk about her physical health.

⇒ The invaluable information given by Mrs. Rivas while responding to the first two questions would not have surfaced had Dr. Chang not used an open-ended approach to initiate the interview.

⇒ After gaining insight into the patient's background, Dr. Chang took note of her mental state and proceeded to ask the third question to inquire about the cause that precipitated the visit. Mrs. Rivas quickly offered answers.

⇒ The information collected by Dr. Chang indicates to him that Mrs. Rivas may be very attached to her cultural values. Although she lives with other family members and is being cared for financially, she has unmet emotional needs subsequent to the death of her husband.

⇒ Dr. Chang may decide to further explore Mrs. Rivas' emotional state by asking her a question that will help her talk about her husband. To learn more about the patient's social support system, Dr. Chang may ask Mrs. Rivas a question about her relationship with her daughter and her family.

Patient 2: Tomás González

Tomás is a twenty-year-old man who is referred by the physician to Mrs. Mahler, the social worker at the community health center.

Mrs. Mahler:	Good morning, Tomás. Come in.
Tomás:	Hi. I'd like to know if you have pamphlets to give away.
Mrs. Mahler:	What kind of pamphlets are you looking for?
Tomás:	Nothing special I guess, just different kinds.
Mrs. Mahler:	O.K., I can get those for you. I see in your file that you may also be in need of some advice.
Tomás:	Well, it's just that the doctor thinks that I should think about doing something about my problem.
Mrs. Mahler:	What is that, Tomás?
Tomás:	Well, my wife and I have a three-year-old daughter. Our daughter was born when we were still in high school. I'm afraid that my wife will get pregnant. I still haven't been able to get us an apartment. We live with her parents and brothers and sisters.
Mrs. Mahler:	Are you using a contraceptive method?
Tomás:	Me? No, of course *I'm* not. She is. She's using the rhythm method because she says that's the only

method the Catholic Church approves, you know? I've told my wife that we need some real protection, but she won't listen to me. She only listens to her mother. I keep telling her we should do what all our friends are doing. We were both born here!

Mrs. Mahler: Is your wife working?

Tomás: No, she has to take care of the baby. I'm working day and night and I still can't make ends meet. I wish we could move into an apartment of our own! My wife always has to help her mother make the tacos and clean the house on weekends and holidays. I usually go out with her brothers to get the beers. We party at home, but sometimes I wish my wife and I could go to a football game instead of partying at home with her family. I'm getting tired of being drunk every weekend!

Using the GREET Approach

Mrs. Mahler listened to Tomás' concerns as he spoke about his problem. She also observed that his facial and body expressions suggested frustration and anger at times.

Generation. Tomás is a second-generation Latino. He is a mainstream American.

Reason. (doesn't apply)

Extended or nuclear family. As a consequence of financial difficulties, Tomás and his wife live with his wife's extended family. Yet, he would prefer to live in a nuclear family setting.

Ethnic behavior. They share Mexican food and music with his wife's family. They celebrate Mexican and U.S. holidays. Frequent family gatherings often lead to drinking heavily.

Time living in the U.S. He has lived in the U.S. all his life. Therefore, his ways are often mainstream.

Key Points

⇒ Mrs. Mahler's questions were intended to make Tomás feel at ease in order to facilitate the encounter. He eagerly offered information.

⇒ Mrs. Mahler understands that Tomás finds himself in conflict between two cultures. He and his wife became teenage parents in high school. Although his ethnic behavior is mostly mainstream, he respects his wife's views. Yet, he does not appear to be willing to use a contraceptive method himself, probably because of machismo. He considers it his wife's responsibility, not his, to prevent a pregnancy. Mrs. Mahler reminds herself that she is dealing with a young Latino couple who are struggling to succeed between two cultures. While Tomás is more individualistic and mainstream in his view of life, his wife is more collectivistic and remains attached to Latino values.

⇒ They live with his wife's extended family, and his mother-in-law provides advice regarding birth control. Although he would like to be independent and go to mainstream recreational activities, his wife seems to be more attached to her family. There appears to be alcohol use in significant amounts on weekend family get-togethers and celebrations.

⇒ Mrs. Mahler may ask Tomás to bring his wife to the office next time he comes. She may want to discuss with the couple the options they have regarding birth control.

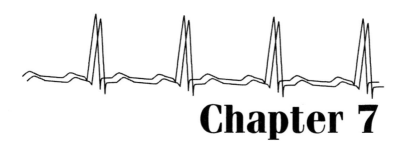

Chapter 7

LISTEN: Gaining Access to Your Patient's Clinical History

Two main difficulties in gaining an accurate patient history arise from the differences in attitude that Latinos and mainstream Americans have toward health and disease. First, Americans are used to giving straight-to-the-point answers when asked about their health history. In contrast, Latinos appear to ramble. They hardly ever respond directly, which can give the impression that they are reluctant to provide complete answers to the clinicians' questions. Second, Americans may bring a mental list of symptoms to report; however, Latino patients often contribute information only when asked. This indirect manner of responding to questions during the medical interview, called *indirectas* (Tirado 1996), can be frustrating to a non-Latino provider because the reason for consultation seems to emerge only at the end of the interview. Understanding the cultural reasons behind this Latino behavior can help the provider overcome these cultural barriers.

There are two cultural explanations for this indirectness. First, as discussed in chapter 1, many immigrants come from countries with paternalistic systems of health care, where the state adopts a protective attitude toward the individual. Thus, in the minds of patients who came from such systems, the responsibility of figuring out what is wrong with them is in the provider's hands. Latino patients consider providers to be very knowledgeable and expect them to be able to diagnose their health problems. For some Latinos, responsibility for personal health may go only as far as reaching the clinician's office and taking the prescribed treatment. In their minds, the provider is responsible for requesting the appropriate information, finding the cause of the problem, and fixing it. In other words being healthy largely comes from having a good health provider.

Second, the fear of having a severe illness may lead the patient to suppress information. This fear is often rooted in the belief that illnesses are caused by bad spirits or by God as a form of punishment. In such a case the patient's fear that bad behavior has brought on illness provokes a fatalistic attitude, leading the patient to believe there is little to be done. When fatalism and religiosity take over in the patient's mind, health is seen as being in the hands of the provider, who, in turn, is guided by God. Latinos may believe that God will determine whether the provider will uncover the true nature of the illness. In other words, a Latino's fear of having an irreversible condition is often overwhelming.

Given these potential difficulties, it is important that you proceed with caution when gathering information for the clinical history. You face the challenge of asking questions that encourage the patient to contribute information while understanding how cultural issues may affect the patient's responses. This chapter will help you gain access to the Latino's clinical history and organize key elements of the interview that emerge from the answers.

The Clinical History

Many providers use a standard format for collecting a patient's clinical history. Some Latino patients may appear uncomfortable when responding to questions that might seem like basic, innocuous information to a mainstream provider. This section describes cultural issues that may arise when a provider is asking for personal information, the cause for consultation, a history of the current health problem, medical history, social history, and family history. It also reveals how even the most standard questions can touch on topics that Latinos consider private or improper.

Personal Data

Most of the questions regarding personal information can be answered with straightforward answers: name, age, and occupation. There is one exception. Sometimes a mother may hesitate to give the last name of an illegitimate child. It is customary to temporarily give an illegitimate child the mother's last name in hopes of changing it to the father's last name in the future. When a mother hesitates about offering a child's last name, the best approach is to move on without causing distress. To inquire about nationality, the best approach is to first ask the patient for his or her place of birth and next about nationality. Place of birth is a neutral item, one which most people are proud of, but questions about nationality may cause discomfort. In the United States people are either citizens or aliens. For some, even the term *resident alien* produces angst because it is perceived to be a step lower than a U.S. citizen. Other Latinos may believe that less respect is accorded to "aliens."

Clinical History of Current Health Problem

Once the provider has identified the patient's reason for seeking health care, obtaining the details of the current health problem is less challenging. However, getting all of the relevant details about the ailment requires practice and patience because, as noted, Latinos seldom give direct answers. When describing the evolution of a health problem, a patient may combine personal interpretations, emotional issues, and cultural health beliefs and practices. Consequently, the provider needs to discern the facts from the patient's interpretations of them and may encounter varying degrees of difficulty understanding the connections between the illness and reasons the patient gives as the cause.

In describing a constant chest pain, for example, an elderly patient might say, "It began the moment I had an argument with my daughter and I got on my knees to pray to the Virgin of Guadalupe for help." The patient might also describe the pain "...as if I had a knife in my chest because that's how my daughter has hurt me." According to the patient, "The pain is only bearable when I drink the tea that the *maestro* (folk healer) gave me." Try to carefully consider everything the patient has said and extract those facts that are relevant to the current ailment. The patient's health beliefs and practices must not be disregarded, because they are part of the patient's reality. Failing to consider the patient's cultural beliefs may result in a patient's lack of commitment to treatment. In fact, the patient's metaphors help illustrate the magnitude of pain and/or suffering he or she is experiencing and the degree of trust placed in the folk healer.

Past Medical History

Latino patients are very good at giving information regarding their past medical histories, and if the patient perceives that you are caring, he or she will often spend a lot of time describing previous ailments in great detail. Hoping to please, the patient may even steer away from the current health problem. In that case, it is always useful to remind the patient that only the relevant information is necessary. Discussing past ailments appears to be easier because it causes less anguish. In contrast, facing current health problems generates uncertainty and fear.

Some adult patients may not clearly recall childhood diseases and immunizations. Since the health of a child is considered to be mainly the mother's responsibility, few people make the effort to actually record this information. Do not judge this lack of knowledge, because, as I have discussed several times, personal responsibility for one's health is not a concept that is familiar to many Latinos.

Few cultural issues related to past surgeries, complications, adult illnesses, immunizations, allergies, or medications will inhibit the patient's responses to medical history questions. There is one exception, though: surgeries or illnesses related to women's reproductive systems. In particular, some women feel that having had a hysterectomy makes them less attractive because they lack reproductive ability. Therefore, they prefer to avoid the subject. Yet, when asked directly, they will often give detailed explanations. Providers should not refrain from asking questions as necessary.

When asking about health habits and diets, the provider may want to keep in mind that although some ethnic foods may not be considered healthy according to U.S. nutritional and dietary standards, they may be ingrained in a patient's culture, much as french fries and hamburgers are in the mainstream American diet. For example, Mexicans enjoy eating fat pork rinds called *chicharrones* while drinking beer, and fried foods are popular among Puerto Ricans and Central Americans. Drinking habits must be carefully investigated in terms of type, quantity, and frequency. For some, drinking a couple of beers is considered a medicinal practice and is not reported as alcohol consumption. For others, heavy alcohol use during holidays is a social activity described by some as "an opportunity to share" with friends and family and is unlikely to be perceived as alcohol abuse. Alcohol abuse may, in fact, be defined differently. For example, among some people of Mexican origin, drinking is mostly considered bad when it gives rise to domestic violence and humiliating scenes that convey lack of respect toward family members.

Social History

Dignity and willpower are two powerful cultural values that are deeply rooted in the collectivistic social life of Latinos, and they strongly influence patients' attitudes toward health and disease. Willpower is one's inner strength, which the individual believes can overcome anything. Dignity is based on having self-respect, which encourages others to respect the individual, a priority for most Latinos. A patient with terminal cancer may seek a dignified end of life by refusing treatment, and a Latino male struggling to overcome alcohol abuse may reject therapy by stating that his willpower will help him get rid of the problem by himself. In both cases the patients' attitudes stem from their cultural values. In contrast, an individualistic mainstream patient may willingly accept chemotherapy to treat cancer or enter a rehabilitation program to overcome an alcohol problem. A provider's understanding of these two underlying but powerful values will increase opportunities to create an effective bridge to communication.

Family History

As discussed in GREET, you may want to consider the patient's age, generation, and level of education when collecting information regarding family history. An elderly patient may not remember details regarding parents' or siblings' health problems unless there is a disease that runs in the family. Children and adolescents often know very little about the health histories of their families. Adults who have lived in the United States for several years, however, often learn how to respond to questions regarding family history and are able to give effective answers. Third-generation Latinos are often bilingual and bicultural; they are highly effective in communicating family history. Belief in and treatment for folk diseases are common among those with lower educational levels, especially if they are monolingual.

Questions Regarding Organs and Systems

In general the more educated or acculturated the patient, the less difficult it will be to approach certain topics. However, there are a number of cultural issues regarding certain organs that make Latino patients uncomfortable and thus reluctant to discuss.

For women three areas fall into this category and should be approached carefully: the gynecological system, the urinary system, and information regarding sexual activity. As discussed in chapter 2, according to the cultural value of marianismo, women are expected to be virtuous and dignified, like the Virgin Mary. The value is so ingrained in the culture that it is customary for some people to describe their mothers or their wives by saying, "My mother is a saint." Therefore, asking a woman if she has had syphilis or gonorrhea is considered disrespectful. When requesting such sensitive information, you may want to say, "Well, I need to ask you this but it's only just in case." If in fact the female patient has a positive answer, no harm has been done. Similarly, if the patient (an immigrant) is elderly and engaged in sexual activity at a young age, it is appropriate to say, "Yes, that's the way it used to be back then." This statement creates a level of comfort for the patient because she feels respected by the provider.

Some Latinas consider the urinary system to be part of their sexual organs; therefore, the same care should be exercised when asking questions about this area of the body. In addition, some less-educated women view their sexual organs as a means of accomplishing their reproductive responsibilities in life. Some may consider sexual activity unnecessary after the children have been born and the family is complete.

Machismo, which influences how Latino men view their masculinity, also affects how providers should approach topics involving sexuality. Sexual activity and sexual organs are two subjects that must be handled carefully by the provider in order to obtain credible responses. Many Latinos exaggerate when they talk about their sexual activity and often brag about their promiscuity. There is a double standard, especially among less-educated Latinos. Although women should be like the Virgin Mary, men can have extramarital or extrarelational affairs because of their machismo. At any rate, there is a rule of thumb among Latino physicians: when men report their sexual activity, divide the number by two.

Also because of their machismo, men are often reluctant to talk about either transitory or permanent impotency. When asking about sexual dysfunction, a useful approach is to say, "Well, has it ever happened to you? It is normal, you know." This statement often offers reassurance and can open the door to important revelations.

LISTEN: Six Key Elements

The second step toward achieving cultural competence with Latinos is LISTEN. It will assist you in overcoming cultural barriers that can present a challenge when you are attempting to gather information for a clinical history. LISTEN will help you uncover the reason that brings the patient to the consultation. The LISTEN acronym stands for

L = Language
I = Illness
S = Subject
T = Touch
E = Educational level
N = Norms of the culture

Language

Linguistic competence is part of an ideal situation, since most non-Latino providers do not speak Spanish and must rely on an intermediary to act as an interpreter. While the intervention of a third person may aid linguistic communication, it may also diminish opportunities to gather information of a private or intimate nature and may prevent some important information from emerging during the encounter. Being aware of this challenge is critical because it prepares you to use your ability to probe and seek answers in creative ways. For example, familiarity with the Spanish terms for common symptoms such as pain, fever, weakness, and so forth will help with a Latino patient who has limited English proficiency. It will usually produce a positive response.

Illness

In most cases the patient seeks biomedical help only after self-care, a folk healer, or both have failed. Under this circumstance, rising anxiety in the patient may lead the patient to believe that something is very wrong. Regardless of the accuracy of the patient's assumption, the perception affects the amount of information the patient will volunteer. For example, a patient who suspects that cancer may be a potential diagnosis of his or her condition may provide limited information out of fear of confirmation. In this case, it is better to drop the subject, continue to build rapport with the patient, and leave the specific questions for the final part of the interview.

Subject

Latinos and Latinas avoid discussing uncomfortable subjects if they believe the matter is irrelevant to the reason for their visit. Therefore, knowing what subjects to avoid is helpful. If sensitive subjects must be discussed, they are always best left for last. Women, especially first-generation immigrants and the elderly, may, as I've just mentioned, become uncomfortable if asked to discuss their sex life. You may want to carefully lead the discussion in that direction and wait for the right moment to ask an indirect question or to suggest the subject. For example, asking a female patient whether she would like to discuss any aspects of her intimate life may open the discussion if the patient is at ease. Men, on the other hand, have few problems discussing most topics except, of course, sexual dysfunction. It is often helpful to ask a man whether there are any aspects of his health that make him unhappy. This question will often trigger the desired answer.

Domestic dysfunction is one topic that both spouses will avoid discussing. Revealing family problems to a stranger is interpreted as a lack of loyalty to the family. In this case, suggesting that children's well-being may be at stake releases the tension and often leads to an open discussion of the problem. Knowing the subjects that are uncomfortable for each gender and age group will help you approach them either indirectly or after all other questions have been asked and the patient is more at ease.

The provider's gender is another important factor in the equation. While women are usually more relaxed with a female provider, men have no preference unless their problem is impotence. Male patients prefer to discuss this subject with a male provider to protect their manliness.

Touch

Placing a hand on the patient's hand can act as a bridge to communication. Whenever you perceive a gap, touch can convey a sense of respect and sensitivity that Latino patients greatly appreciate. It is culturally acceptable for a female or male provider to touch a female patient's hand briefly. However, a male or a female provider would normally not place a hand on a male patient unless the patient is elderly or is crying.

Educational Level

In general the more educated the patient, the easier it will be to obtain key information. The health beliefs of well-educated patients tend to reflect the biomedical model of disease. Such patients describe symptoms and signs readily and ask meaningful questions. Patients with low educational levels, however, may present more of a challenge. While describing their symptoms, they may also offer their opinion regarding causation according to their health beliefs. These explanations may help you uncover important additional information and therefore should not be ignored.

For example, an immigrant Mexican mother may initially rate her son's health as excellent. After you probe with a question like "Anything else about the baby's first years?" however, she may add that the only times her son was in the hospital were when the boy developed mollera caída. (See chapter 3 for more information.) You might learn that according to the mother, the nurse who examined the child's anterior fontanelle was the cause of the problem. In reality, the child may have had a long history of repetitive hospitalizations due to dehydration as a consequence of his lactose intolerance.

The fear of having cancer, however, may build a wall of resistance during the interview, regardless of the patient's educational level. A patient who appears reticent, anxious, and fearful may be hiding such a concern. If you suspect this to be the case, you may find it useful to probe carefully and ask questions that lead to more detailed descriptions. Follow-up questions such as "Can you describe more?" "How so?" and "What exactly do you mean by that?" generally encourage the patient to continue describing the problem. For example, a patient who admits to having problems with bowel movements may, with additional probing, admit to passing blood, having significant weight loss, and even adding that colon cancer "runs in the family."

Norms of the Culture

Two cultural norms especially influence the history-taking aspect of the clinical encounter. First, familism is a critical aspect. Because Latinos are strongly collectivistic (Lecca et al. 1998), a sickness affects all family members and not just the individual who is ill. Therefore, patients often come to seek help accompanied by one or more family members who are there to provide transportation, interpretation, or moral support. While the relatives' presence may sometimes appear to make the interview more difficult, family members often contribute valuable information. In fact, some family members accompany the patient with the purpose of supplying information that the patient may be reluctant to provide. In this case, the patient will not resent the relative's intervention. For example, while a husband may report that he eats a low-fat diet at home, the wife may add that he often cheats when he is away from home. The accompanying relatives often assume the active role while the sick patient remains passive. For example, the sick spouse often delegates the talking to the accompanying spouse, the mother speaks for the child, or a daughter may speak for her elderly mother.

Second, patients need the provider's reassurance of respect (familism and respect are discussed in chapter 2). One way to convey respect is to use the proper titles to address the patient. Most non-Latino providers who speak Spanish use *Usted* as a general rule and with very good results (for a discussion of titles, see pages 98–99). Having a nonjudgmental attitude to-

ward the patient's health beliefs and practices also helps
to convey respect during the history taking. This can
be attained by abstaining from exhibiting any facial
reaction when the patient candidly explains the meaning of symptoms or the type of health-seeking behavior sought. In sum, understanding the norms of the
culture is critical in the assessment of the clinical history.

LISTEN in Practice

The next two vignettes illustrate the use of the LIS-
TEN approach by two providers. The discussion at
the end of each vignette presents the critical points
that the LISTEN approach highlights.

Patient 1: Roberto Martinez

The patient, a fifty-year-old, first-generation male of
Central American origin, migrated from Nicaragua
eight years ago and works as a supervisor of a construction crew. He is a high school graduate with vocational training. Rose Watson, a nurse working in the
emergency room, greets Mr. Martinez (she earlier observed that his wife was in the waiting room).

Mrs. Watson:	Good evening, Señor Martinez. Please come in and have a seat. (She shakes hands with the patient and smiles.)
Mr. Martinez:	Thank you. I thought I was going to have a male doctor see me. I asked for one.

Mrs. Watson: I'm aware of that, Señor Martinez, but right now I'm the only one who is available to help you. What brings you to the emergency room at this time of the night?

Mr. Martinez: Well, I work very hard every day. I'm in charge of a crew and it's a big responsibility. I can't come during the day.

Mrs. Watson: Did something happen that made you come tonight?

Mr. Martinez: Well, yes. Even if I had wanted to, I couldn't have come earlier because I had to work overtime as usual. I got home at nine-thirty and had dinner at ten. I hadn't even had a chance to take a break or have a soda all day today. I have a big problem.

Mrs. Watson: And how can I help you? (She briefly makes eye contact with Mr. Martinez.)

Mr. Martinez: Tonight I went to the bathroom to defecate. I noticed there was blood in the toilet bowl.

Mrs. Watson: I see.... Can you describe the color of the blood?

Mr. Martinez: It was bright red. God, it was so scary.

Mrs. Watson:	I understand what you mean. How much did you bleed? (She makes brief eye contact again.)
Mr. Martinez:	I don't remember; everything in the toilet bowl looked like blood to me. I panicked.
Mrs. Watson:	Señor Martinez, how long has this problem been going on?
Mr. Martinez:	I don't know, maybe for a week. I'm not sure.
Mrs. Watson:	So tonight wasn't the first time.
Mr. Martinez:	I guess not. Do you think I have cancer?
Mrs. Watson:	We'll take one step at a time, Señor Martinez. In order to help you, I need to have all the details regarding the problem. Would you like for me to call your wife so she can help you? (She responds in a calm and reassuring tone.)

Using the LISTEN Approach

Language. Language is not a barrier to communication. Mr. Martinez is fluent in English. However, Mr. Martinez makes use of a number of indirect statements out of fear of cancer.

Illness. For Mr. Martinez, as for other Latinos, blood, cancer, and death are often viewed as a triad. In his mind he has cancer. When Mrs. Watson asks questions, the patient is too upset to give direct answers and is using Latino indirectness. The terrifying thought of having cancer prevents him from supplying relevant information. Mrs. Watson realizes that the patient is roaming because of his extreme anxiety. She adopts a supportive attitude and refers to the bleeding neutrally as "the problem" in order to help the patient talk about it more easily. She calmly suggests they take one step at a time.

Subject. Latino men prefer to talk about health problems dealing with private body parts and private bodily functions with male providers. Therefore, the patient is uncomfortable talking to a female nurse. Mrs. Watson makes special efforts to project a professional image to help the patient ignore the fact that he is talking to a female provider. She shakes his hand initially and subsequently makes eye contact briefly when Mr. Martinez describes the blood he passed.

Touch. Because the patient is male, Mrs. Watson abstains from placing her hand on Mr. Martinez because it would be inappropriate. However, she makes eye contact often, speaks with a reassuring voice, and maintains a tone of voice that conveys respect and empathy toward his ordeal.

Educational Level. Mr. Martinez is a high school graduate and has vocational training. He has also received training on his job. This helps him to be articulate and able to communicate verbally. Yet, there are cultural barriers in the encounter. For example, Mr. Martinez is not fully at ease with a female provider. Aware of this, Mrs. Watson offers to ask the patient's wife to join them in her office, hoping that the patient's wife may be able to complement the information given by her husband.

Norms of the Culture. Mrs. Watson is aware of the fact that Mr. Martinez was accompanied to the hospital by his wife, who may have come for the purpose of providing complementary information or to adopt an active role in view of the nature of her husband's illness. Mrs. Watson suspects that Mr. Martinez' wife may help confirm his version of the problem and may even supply additional details regarding his eating habits. Mrs. Watson suspects that the patient may be downplaying the magnitude of the symptoms and signs. She is also careful to always address the patient as "Señor Martinez."

Key Points

⇛ Mrs. Watson found out through questioning Mrs. Martinez that Mr. Martinez had a ten-year history of constipation and hemorrhoids. Due to a pressing work schedule, he had not been careful about his diet lately. The patient had recently been promoted to supervisor and was very focused on becoming his company's best employee. His constipation exacerbated the problem with his hemorrhoids. He hadn't been drinking enough fluids or eating properly and hadn't had time to use the bathroom regularly. These factors accentuated his constipation problem. This was his first incident with profusely bleeding hemorrhoids.

⇛ Mr. Martinez' wife may potentially act as the bridge of communication between him and Mrs. Watson.

Patient 2: María Moreno

María Moreno is a forty-five-year-old Latina from Puerto Rico who is experiencing marital problems with her husband. Mrs. Jones, a licensed clinical psychologist, interviews her for the first time. After María spends five minutes talking generally about the family, Mrs. Jones presses and asks more direct questions.

Mrs. Jones:	Would you like to tell me a bit about your life with your husband?
Mrs. Moreno:	Well, we used to be so happy when we got married, but that was a long time ago. I got pregnant when I was in junior high and had to drop out of school. But it did not matter; we were so in love, so happy. So many things are not the same anymore.
Mrs. Jones:	What has changed?
Mrs. Moreno:	He used to be so romantic. We used to make love all the time. But then, well, the children came, and there are so many responsibilities now.
Mrs. Jones:	Did something happen to make things different?
Mrs. Moreno:	You see, there was so much passion in our life back in Puerto Rico. After we moved to the U.S., there wasn't time for that anymore. He's always in a hurry and

	we're both so tired all the time. He always complains that I'm tired. The children need me more than he does, I think.
Mrs. Jones:	Have you talked about this with your husband?
Mrs. Moreno:	Oh, yes. But he's always complaining about me. He says I've become cold.
Mrs. Jones:	Do you think you have, María?
Mrs. Moreno:	No. He never brings me flowers anymore and he knows I'm very sentimental. He forgets my birthdays and our anniversaries. All he wants is sex. He says that a neighbor put a curse on us. I went to see Dona, an espiritista who works in our community, and she confirmed it. She said there is a neighbor who is trying to steal my husband from me. She gave me some treatment for both of us.
Mrs. Jones:	Did it work?
Mrs. Moreno:	Well, a little, but I'm still using it. My husband refuses to drink it. So I decided to come to you to see if you can also help. I think that I've fulfilled my duty by becoming a mother three times. Now I have to take care of our children, but my husband doesn't understand that. I'm afraid he'll leave me because

the other woman can make him happy and I can't. (Mrs. Moreno starts crying.)

Mrs. Jones: I'm sorry. I'm sure that you are also concerned about the children. Do they know that you and your husband are having problems?

Mrs. Moreno: Yes, I'm afraid they do. It breaks my heart to see my oldest daughter crying.

Mrs. Jones: I can imagine what you must be going through. (She briefly puts her hand on Mrs. Moreno's hand as she hands her a tissue.)

Mrs. Moreno: Do you think you can help?

Mrs. Jones: I'll do my best. We have a team here that can work with you. Do you think that your husband would be willing to come with you to our next session? It is important for him to also get involved in finding a solution to the problem.

Mrs. Moreno: I think he will come if I tell him that you asked that he come. He'll be upset at first because I told you about our problems. But he'll get over it, and he'll do it for our children. He'll come with me next time. He has to do it for our family.

Using the LISTEN Approach

Language. Although language is not a barrier to communication between Mrs. Moreno and Mrs. Jones, Mrs. Jones forms her sentences and questions carefully to avoid idiomatic expressions and difficult grammar construction. Also, several issues around familism challenged Mrs. Jones' cultural competence skills. First, she asked questions about the family to convey the message that she was not only interested in the patient but also in her family's well-being. Next, without being aggressive, she carefully framed the questions to allow the patient to make the decision to discuss private matters with ease. This was critical to getting Mrs. Moreno to disclose private family matters to a stranger. Finally, when the patient opened up, Mrs. Jones began calling the patient by her first name, which created a sense of intimacy. Being a woman provider was an added asset in an interview with a female patient, especially considering the delicate issues involved.

Illness. In Mrs. Moreno's mind, her marital problems were a curse, and she was looking for help to supplement the espiritista's treatment. Mrs. Jones used the neutral word *problem* so as not to conflict with the couple's belief that there might be a curse on them. In the patient's mind, the cause of her and her husband's marital difficulties was supernatural.

Subject. For the patient, discussing intimate aspects of her marriage was difficult. Yet, she overcame her reluctance because Mrs. Jones took five minutes to get to know her as a person and because she believed she needed to find a confidant. A female provider seemed like a good opportunity.

Touch. During the interview Mrs. Jones placed her hand on Mrs. Moreno's hand to show support.

Educational Level. The patient had only finished junior high school in Puerto Rico. Her health beliefs and behaviors matched her level of education.

Norms of the Culture. Mrs. Jones considered the norms of María's culture and tried to avoid being judgmental. Instead, she actively listened to her patient. She understood that María's reality revolved around her husband, her children, and her espiritista. María's marianismo and her husband's machismo clearly tinted her life's vision.

Key Points

⇒ Mrs. Jones understood she had to be sensitive toward Mrs. Moreno's cultural beliefs regarding the cause of the problem. To show her sensitivity, Mrs. Jones chose not to ignore or belittle the patient's belief in the espiritista's powers. She also did not try to compete with the espiritista.

⇒ Mrs. Jones realized that culture had a tremendous impact on Mrs. Moreno's views on marriage and the family. Mrs. Jones conveyed concern about the potential consequences of domestic problems on her children. María confirmed that her children's well-being was her priority at the moment.

⇒ Mrs. Jones suggested that Mrs. Morreno come to the next appointment with her husband.

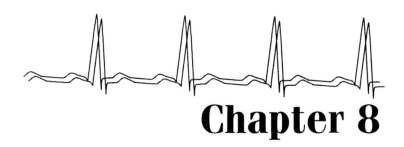

Chapter 8

CARE: Performing a Culturally Sensitive Patient Evaluation

The Culturally Competent Physical Examination

The purpose of this chapter is to use the CARE approach to highlight aspects that may help providers perform a culturally sensitive physical and/or mental health evaluation. Latinos bring a myriad of expectations to the physical examination. Many perceive the American medical system as focused on the procedure more than on the patient. Despite this perception, they hope to find a provider who can connect at a personal level, who will ask for their permission to be examined before the procedure begins, and who will explain each step of the exam as it progresses. When the personal touch is absent, the Latino patient's apprehensiveness is often evident in his or her facial expression, nervousness, and posture. Needless to say, in such cases, the communication breaks down between patient and provider.

There are two particular areas of concern for Latinos when they are being examined. First, they have specific cultural expectations about how the provider carries out the exam. For example, patients hope that the provider will keep private parts of the body covered at all times except during the examination of those areas. Second, there are issues of respect associated with particular parts of the body. Understanding a Latino patient's perspective can be extremely helpful in getting the cooperation of the patient during the exam. For example, asking the patient to expose the area to be examined instead of uncovering it yourself works best. In addition, a culturally sensitive examination significantly increases the quality of care the provider can offer.

Latinos in general place a great deal of importance on the privacy of certain parts of their body. Furthermore, there are differences between how Latinos and mainstream Americans define "private parts." For example, even the lower part of the neck and the back may be private for some Latinos. For many, thighs and hips are not to be exposed publicly. For most, breasts and genital areas are private parts. As a rule of thumb, any part of the body that is normally covered with clothing is potentially a private part, although each individual reacts differently. Therefore, the culturally appropriate behavior when performing the physical examination consists of presenting a friendly yet formal attitude, identifying the patient's personal issues, and responding to them effectively and respectfully.

Examining Patients of Different Age and Gender

Latino patients' perceptions of the body vary depending on age and gender. Based on modesty issues, men, women, children, and the elderly have different areas of concern regarding physical examinations. In general, less acculturated individuals have more concerns than more acculturated and second-generation Latinos. This section explains the particularities of carrying out a physical examination with different age and gender groups.

Children. A child usually communicates with the provider through the parent. At least one parent generally accompanies a preadolescent to the provider's office, provides the information for the clinical history, and is present during the physical examination. The parent's presence is reassuring to the child. For example, during an abdominal palpation, the child may be more willing to contribute information regarding discomfort or pain to the parent rather than to the clinician. Therefore, unless there is a reason to examine the child without the parent being present, it is usually helpful to have the parent's assistance.

Youth. Latino teenagers, like American mainstream teens, are often independent and prefer to be examined without the parent being present. While young males may appear to be comfortable, young female patients often appear to have modesty issues that require a tactful and understanding exam. For example, before subjecting a teenage Latina to a vaginal examination, you may first opt to draw a diagram or show a picture to the patient to help explain the exam and discuss its importance. Knowing what to expect (discomfort, pressure, mild pain, etc.) may help distract her attention away from modesty concerns. Suggesting that the presence of the mother or accompanying female relative is welcome in the office may help ease the anxiety in the female patient.

Women. The physical exam is an unpleasant experience for many women (Martinez et al. 1997). Those who have had children are less modest, but unmarried women who, according to cultural norms, are not supposed to have an active sexual life before marriage, appear to struggle with exposing the body during the exam. They are more at ease with female clinicians and have more modesty issues when examined by a male provider.

For most Latinas, married or unmarried, the examination of the breasts and the genital, vaginal, and rectal areas demands that you be tactful and perform the examination in the least possible time regardless of whether the provider is a male or female. While most unmarried women do not welcome a pelvic exam, married women accept it as part of being in their reproductive years. A vaginal exam should only be performed on a woman after explaining the exam and subsequent to obtaining the consent of the patient if she is an adult or of the accompanying parent if the patient is a minor. Only the area of the body under examination should be exposed while the rest of the body remains covered. Women especially appreciate explanations of each step as the exam proceeds.

Men. Most male Latinos accept a physical examination without anxiety. For some, though, exposing the genital area produces discomfort regardless of the gender of the provider. Thus, the area should be exposed only when carrying out the exam. Aside from those who are well endowed, Latino males are shy about exposing their penises and will often cover them with one hand while the clinician is examining neighboring areas.

Because of machismo, some Latino men may reject a rectal examination because it is linked with the loss of manliness. Some believe that only gay men accept penetration of the rectal area. Therefore, you will want to ask the patient's permission to perform the exam. If permission is granted, the exam should be carried out tactfully, efficiently, and promptly. If the patient refuses the exam, go on with the evaluation and bring up the subject later and explain why the exam is important.

Elderly Patients. The majority of elderly Latinos are foreign-born immigrants who, despite the number of years they have lived in the United States, still retain many of their cultural health beliefs. In particular, they like to discuss their concerns about their blood pressure, cholesterol, and blood sugar count. When they seek health care, they often have either a chronic condition or a health concern caused by a recent onset of disturbing signs or symptoms. In either case it is possible that they have not had a physical exam in years, so in most cases they welcome one.

Elderly women may, however, strongly reject and resent a vaginal, pelvic, or rectal exam. They believe that after having lived through their reproductive years, they do not need to have those areas of their bodies examined. Elderly men, on the other hand, usually have no concerns regarding a physical examination and even accept a rectal exam stoically.

CARE and the Physical Examination

The purpose of the CARE approach is to facilitate the procedures of a standard physical exam. This step encompasses the cultural issues that you may want to consider when attempting to carry out a culturally sensitive physical exam.

Four critical aspects are especially important when examining a Latino or a Latina patient.

C = Cover the body
Λ = Attention
R = Respect
E = Eye contact

Cover the Body

Latinos and Latinas are generally modest. They welcome the robes or sheets provided to cover their bodies before and during a physical examination. They also prefer that you ask them to expose the area of the body to be examined while they keep the rest of their bodies covered. There are differences in male and female attitudes toward exposing the body. Except for the genital area, men tend to show no concern about exposing their bodies. Women, however, are, as mentioned earlier, very timid about exposing their bodies. In order to better respond to these sentiments, ask for permission to examine the body and, after examining each area, you may suggest that the patient replace the cover. Should a patient refuse to uncover her body, you should explain the importance of the exam in making a successful diagnosis. Should the patient continue to refuse the exam, you may offer other options such as deferring the exam for a subsequent appointment or referring the patient to another provider.

Attention

A Latino patient expects your undivided attention during the physical exam. The patient often observes your facial expressions closely to confirm that you are paying attention to each step of the exam. Showing a distracted demeanor or allowing outside interruptions while performing a physical examination will interfere with establishing a satisfactory patient-provider relationship. For example, a Latino patient would consider your responding to a knock on the door or to a telephone call an extremely disrespectful act unless the reason for the interruption is an extreme emergency. On the other hand, Latinos often welcome the presence of interns; they do not generally present an inconvenience because Latinos consider interns as doctors-in-training who are collaborating in improving their health. Patients often tell their relatives that a team of doctors participated in their recovery.

Respect

Respect is a central value of Latino culture (see chapter 2 for a discussion), and it is very important that care be taken to show respect to the patient during a physical examination. During the inspection, palpation, percussion, and auscultation of the body, the Latino or Latina patient will be sensitive to your reactions toward expressed discomfort, pain, and modesty. Failure to acknowledge the patient's reactions is perceived as a lack of respect.

Discomfort, pain, and modesty may arise during the examination of genital areas in both men and women. In addition to being ill at ease with exposing the genital area, women often express discomfort at merely feeling the contact of a provider's hands. When pain is present, the examination must be carried out diligently but should be ended as promptly as possible. All of these behaviors convey your respect and are highly appreciated by patients. Moreover, explaining the reasons for the exam helps ease the tension. Stop the procedure when the patient reports pain and explain that the exam, although uncomfortable, is necessary. The patient will often report that he or she is "in the hands" of a caring provider.

For women, respect is associated with modesty and virginity. In particular, those who have not initiated sexual activity or who come from rural areas are extremely modest. Virginity is a critical issue for women of any age who are not sexually active. Acknowledging these issues is perceived as respectful.

Eye Contact

Establishing eye contact with the patient is essential, especially when carrying out palpation of areas of the body. The patient will appreciate eye contact, particularly when the provider is checking for painful points. It will reassure the patient that you are attentive, focused on the procedure, and connected with the patient. During the examination of the genital areas, however, eye contact should be made briefly if at all as a sign of respect for the patient's modesty.

CARE in Practice:
The Physical Examination

The following vignettes describe providers using the CARE approach to conduct culturally appropriate physical examinations.

Patient 1: Francisco Cortés

Francisco Cortés is a thirty-five-year-old mechanic who seeks medical attention at a county hospital. He complains of pain during urination and of a feeling of heaviness in his lower abdomen. Chris Yates, a resident physician, evaluates the patient in the emergency room.

Dr. Yates:	Hello, Señor Cortés, I'm Dr. Yates, the resident urologist. I understand you have a problem urinating.
Mr. Cortés:	I do.
Dr. Yates:	I need to examine you, Señor Cortés, if that's O.K. with you.
Mr. Cortés:	O.K. What are you going to do?
Dr. Yates:	Well, I need to check your abdomen and your genital area, and I may have to perform a rectal exam.
Mr. Cortés:	Oh, O.K.
Dr. Yates:	Please expose your abdomen. Does it hurt when I press here? How about here? (He makes brief eye contact with his patient.)
Mr. Cortés:	Yes, it's very tender, especially in the lower part of my belly.
Dr. Yates:	O.K. Now let's take a look at your genital area. Can you please remove the sheet? Do you have a burning sensation when you pass urine? Now, turn over please. I'm going to perform a rectal exam. (There is a knock on Dr. Yates' office door; he ignores it.)
Mr. Cortés:	Is that necessary? I mean, the rectal? (he says reluctantly)
Dr. Yates:	Absolutely. It will be uncomfortable, but we'll be done before you realize it.
Mr. Cortés:	Well, I guess if you have to, you have to. But please don't tell my wife about it.

Dr. Yates: No problem, man. I know what you
              mean. (Dr. Yates looks away as he
              says this.)

Using the CARE Approach

Cover the Body. Dr. Yates is aware of Mr. Cortés' modesty. Before performing the physical evaluation, he asks the patient's permission. He also asks the patient to uncover private parts. This helps Mr. Cortés feel a little more in control and dignified.

Attention. Mr. Cortés follows each step of the physical examination and confirms that Dr. Yates is focused on doing his job thoroughly. When somebody knocks on the door, Dr. Yates ignores it and continues the exam. After this, Mr. Cortés relaxes a bit, thinking that the doctor is concentrating on examining him.

Respect. Dr. Yates shows respect by addressing the patient as Señor Cortés. In addition, he displays sensitivity to Mr. Cortés' machismo by agreeing not to mention the rectal exam to the patient's wife.

Eye Contact. While speaking to the patient, Dr. Yates maintains eye contact. Making eye contact, he performs the abdominal exam and acknowledges Mr. Cortés' painful reactions. He leaves the rectal exam for last and refrains from making eye contact immediately before and after performing it, to save the patient's dignity.

Key Points

⇒ Dr. Yates anticipated Mr. Cortés' bias against having a rectal exam. He mentioned it last when he described to the patient the steps of the examination he was going to perform, trying not to make a big deal about it.

⇒ At the end, he addressed the patient as "man" to reassure him of their mutual manliness, thus respecting Mr. Cortés' machismo.

Patient 2: Iris González

This second vignette illustrates common modesty issues that arise during the physical examination of a young woman.

Iris González is a seventeen-year-old high school student who, with her family, emigrated from El Salvador to the United States ten years ago. Although she has lived most of her life in the country and is perfectly bilingual, she has grown up in a protected environment with her parents. She seeks medical attention because of irregularities with her period. Her mother accompanies her to the doctor's office. She meets her primary care physician, Dr. José Ramos, for the first time.

Dr. Ramos:	Hello, Miss González, I'm Dr. Ramos. Hello, Señora Gonzalez. (He greets the patient and her mother and shakes hands with both.)
Miss González:	Hi, Dr. Ramos. Nice to meet you. I'm glad you're a Latino (she says in a friendly tone).
Dr. Ramos:	Well, I hate to disappoint you, but I was born and raised in

	Texas and I speak very little Spanish. When I was little, my parents moved to the Midwest. All my friends there were Anglo, so I lost my Spanish, much to my mother's disappointment.
Mrs. González:	Oh, that's too bad!
Dr. Ramos:	I know. But I do love Mexican food. Tell me, what brings you here today? (he asks, making eye contact with his patient)
Miss González:	I've been having irregularities with my period.
Mrs. González:	My daughter is a virgin.
Dr. Ramos:	I see. And when was the last time you had your period? (He continues addressing his patient.)
Mrs. González:	She's never had a real physical examination, you know what I mean? Well, maybe she should tell you herself.
Dr. Ramos:	You are right about that, Señora González. Would you like to wait outside while I talk with your daughter?
Mrs. González:	Well, I would prefer to stay here if you don't mind. She's a señorita, you know?
Miss González:	Mama, just go outside and wait for me. It's fine. (Her mother

	reluctantly leaves the doctor's office. The daughter turns to the physician and explains) I had my period two months ago.
Dr. Ramos:	Anything different about that period?
Miss González:	No, well, maybe a lot of cramps, but it wasn't so bad.
Dr. Ramos:	Do you have any idea why you've missed two periods? (He asks the question and makes eye contact with his patient.)
Miss González:	Not really. (She is visibly uncomfortable with the conversation.)
Dr. Ramos:	Do you have a boyfriend?
Miss González:	If you are trying to find out whether I'm having sex, I can answer that. I'm not. I'm a virgin. I've never had a thorough physical and I'm terrified.
Dr. Ramos:	I understand, that's normal. I'm going to examine you but first let me show you a picture of the female reproductive system so I can explain the pelvic exam to you. (He takes out a book and explains the examination that he is about to perform.)
Miss González:	Will it hurt, considering that I have not had sex yet?

Dr. Ramos:	It will be uncomfortable, but it should not hurt. If it does, I want you to let me know. Let me get my assistant, Heidi, in here so she can help. (He calls her on the intercom, and Heidi helps Miss González get ready for the exam.)
Miss González:	I'm so embarrassed. This is the first time I go through this kind of exam (She says this as Dr. Ramos, assisted by Heidi, commences the evaluation.)
Dr. Ramos:	Please tell me if it hurts (he says, while making eye contact with his patient and making sure that her legs are covered).
Miss González:	It hurts a bit but it's not so bad. What's bad is this position; I'm really embarrassed.
Dr. Ramos:	I know what you mean. We're almost done. Everything appears normal. Let's take a Pap smear now. (A few minutes pass.) O.K., Miss González, the exam is over! Please get dressed and come to my office next door so we can talk, O.K.?

Using the CARE Approach

Cover the Body. Dr. Ramos understands that Miss González is making an effort to behave in a mature way and to cooperate with the exam. He tries to be reassuring, and he also uses a picture and explains the exam prior to carrying it out. While examining Miss González, he makes sure the covers stay over her legs at all times while exposing the genital area for access.

Attention. Dr. Ramos focuses on the exam and explains each step so that he can convey to Miss González that he is concentrating on the examination.

Respect. At all times, Dr. Ramos addresses his patient as "Miss González" as a sign of respect and also asks her to let him know if she feels pain. Miss González perceives that the physician respects her feelings and cares about her well-being.

Eye Contact. While performing the most difficult parts of the examination, Dr. Ramos makes eye contact with his patient in a reassuring way.

Key Points

⇒ Dr. Ramos realizes that Señora González has an overprotective attitude and may interfere with the examination. Thus, he courteously asks her if she would like to wait outside. Despite her modesty, Miss González understands the mainstream culture and encourages her mother to leave the office.

⇒ Dr. Ramos is aware of Miss González' modesty; yet he overcomes those feelings by explaining the steps of the exam prior to performing it and by showing her a diagram and having a reassuring and respectful attitude.

The Culturally Competent Mental Health Evaluation

A provider who refers a Latino patient to a mental health professional is often sending a message that the family may perceive as catastrophic. The need for a mental health professional may suggest problems of a serious nature. In fact, complying with numerous appointments may disrupt family dynamics and alter job commitments of family members. In addition, while some Latinos—Puerto Ricans in particular—may link mental illnesses to supernatural causes, others may fear the social stigma that may befall the family. The existence of mental disorders in a family has been known to cause its members to alienate the afflicted person from their social support network. Therefore, it is often useful to begin by suggesting the need for an evaluation "to determine if, in fact, treatment is needed" and by reassuring the family that "things will be dealt with step-by-step." This explanation helps relieve some of the tension in the family.

Evaluating Mental Health

As with the physical examination, the mental health evaluation of a Latino patient should be carried out while keeping the issues of age and gender in mind. Here, though, I also add generation.

Age. In the collectivist Latino culture, adults, usually women, are responsible for caring for the young and the elderly members of the family, as I've discussed earlier. Therefore, children and the elderly rely heavily on the adult woman in the family. For this reason it is not uncommon to find young children and grandparents who appear to be disoriented with respect to time and space.

When contrasted with mainstream American mothers, who encourage independence in their children, immigrant Latino mothers may seem overprotective of their children. They take their children to school and pick them up after class. Younger children may not be able to state their address or have adequate time or space orientation because they are so dependent on their mothers. Older children may also appear to be more passive and reactive than mainstream children because, out of respect, they may rely on their parents to make decisions related to school and friends. Some parents may encourage preteens not to have friends out of fear of drugs in school. Such parents generally emphasize and reward obedience in their children. Thus, children who may appear to have less developed social skills as compared with their peers may in fact have highly active social lives with brothers, sisters, and cousins at home.

Elderly members of the family generally give up their responsibilities and independence and expect their adult children to provide for every aspect of their care. Therefore, they may lose much of their time and space orientation. Nonetheless, there are ways of separating clinical from cultural issues. For example, while some elderly Latinos may not know what day of the month or what year it is, they may clearly recall that the lottery plays on Wednesdays and Saturdays. Similarly, an inability to state an address correctly should not be taken as lack of memory; it is simply a fact that elderly Latinos don't need to know certain things as long as their children are in charge, and the information is even less important to them if they are monolingual.

Gender. As discussed extensively, Latino women and men are influenced by marianismo and machismo, and these roles in turn shape their social behavior. For example, a Latino wife is expected to be submissive to her husband in varying degrees, depending on her level of education. Men are supposed to be strong-willed and to have a high degree of self-assurance because they are the providers for the family. Not being able to fulfill these expected gender roles may trigger emotional distress among Latino couples. In other words, in the view of many Latinos, a woman who is not capable of cooking, cleaning the house, and looking after her children on a day-to-day basis because of a mental condition is not fulfilling her role as the manager of her household, a function attributed to her through marianismo. Likewise, a man who is unemployed and therefore unable to provide for his family lacks machismo because he is not fulfilling his duty.

Generation. Latinos give a great deal of respect to the elderly. At times even second-generation Latinos hesitate to provide information that they feel may damage the special place held by elderly members. In contrast, third-generation Latinos are often critical of their parents' habits and practices. For example, a second-generation individual may easily remember having been given chamomile tea to alleviate an upset stomach during childhood. Thus, if an elderly parent still uses the remedy, the son or daughter can relate to its use. On the other hand, a third-generation mainstream grandchild may not have a clue about the supposed healing properties of chamomile and may regard it as a useless old wives' tale when describing the grandparents' home remedies to the provider.

CARE and the Mental Health Evaluation

Cover the Family

Given the social stigma that Latinos may attach to mental illness, it is important to cover the family's pride. The family will often say that they are bringing their family member because the person is "suffering from nerves." Patients appreciate a provider who initially listens and refrains from aggressively requesting family information. Latinos are often reluctant to reveal to strangers sensitive information pertaining to family dynamics or personal issues of family members. In fact disclosing private information may be considered an act of disloyalty. Therefore, the most effective use of the first appointment is to establish adequate rapport with the patient and family members. You may do this by revealing a few items about yourself. For example, you may say, "I've been to Mexico City but I've never visited Guadalajara" or "I also have a teenage son." The statement may offer the opportunity to start a conversation. Other neutral subjects that may help establish a connection with the patient as well as with the patient's accompanying relatives include food, sports events, and music.

Attention

It is critical to pay equal attention to all family members that come to the initial interview because some will be present only at this interview. You can, through skillful questions to family members, identify key elements of family dynamics that may not be present later. For example, conflicts among family members may surface, or parents may display indifference or emotional outbursts while the patient adopts a passive or aggressive attitude. Once the family members have shown their concern and have assessed and approved of you, they will divert attention toward the patient.

In subsequent interviews, you will have the opportunity to focus attention on and bond with the patient. Using a relatively unstructured approach, interjecting indirect questions, and waiting for the patient to open up will be effective techniques. Very often patients may make reference to apparently unrelated health problems to initiate the disclosure of their emotional problems. For example, a patient may complain of intense headaches that lead to crying. Acknowledging the patient's emotional state often helps. For example, you may comment, "Do you think that something is making you unhappy?" This in turn may trigger an outburst on the patient's part.

Respect

Respect toward religious beliefs and health practices is critical. The patient may have consulted a priest or a folk healer before seeking help from a mental health professional. Some Latinos may believe that their "suffering from nerves" is a consequence of God's punishment for bad deeds; they may be suffering from a great deal of guilt. The best way to show respect is to avoid statements that may suggest criticism or judgment. Instead, encouraging the patient to continue talking will create a respectful atmosphere.

It is wise to always address a patient by his or her last name preceded by a title, as discussed elsewhere. The patient and family will perceive that you respect them. In addition you should create power distance (see chapter 2), which in turn will establish the patient's respect for you. This professional attitude will later encourage greater compliance with a treatment plan. Too much familiarity, on the other hand, may lead family members to perceive you as unprofessional; it may even lead the patient to think you are disrespectful.

Eye Contact

Most patients welcome eye contact because it helps develop closeness to the provider on a personal basis. Eye contact also conveys interest and attention. There is one exception, though. If the patient is struggling to express emotions or is on the verge of disclosing critical information, avoiding eye contact temporarily may help release tension and encourage the patient to talk. It is best to remember, though, that Latinos are a very emotional people, and they appreciate personal attention.

CARE in Practice: The Mental Health Evaluation

The following vignette describes a provider using the CARE approach to conduct a culturally appropriate mental health evaluation.

Patient 3: Aida Real

Mrs. Aida Real, who is seventy years old and of Cuban origin, was found walking alone in a mall. Mrs. Real could not remember where she lived. Paramedics brought her to the emergency room in the early afternoon. Mrs. Tran-Vu, the mental health nurse, was called to evaluate the patient.

Mrs. Tran-Vu:	Hello, can you tell me your full name please? (Mrs. Tran-Vu smiles as she shakes the patient's hand.)
Mrs. Real:	Aida Real.
Mrs. Tran-Vu:	Do you remember what happened to you this morning, Señora Real? (Mrs. Tran-Vu asks, making eye contact.)
Mrs. Real:	Yes, I do. But I don't want to talk about it. (As she says this, she is looking away.)
Mrs. Tran-Vu:	Was there something that happened this morning?

Mrs. Real:	Of course, otherwise I wouldn't be here! (She says this in an irritated manner.)
Mrs. Tran-Vu:	Would you like for me to call your relatives? (She touches the patient's hand as she says this.)
Mrs. Real:	No, thank you. God is going to punish my daughter for being so careless. I don't remember the phone number anyway. But I appreciate your kindness.
Mrs. Tran-Vu:	Do you remember what day of the week it is?
Mrs. Real:	Not really, I don't keep track of that anymore. Well, maybe it's Tuesday, but I'm not sure. Did the lottery play yesterday?
Mrs. Tran-Vu:	No, I don't think so. Would you mind giving me your address? (Mrs. Tran-Vu establishes eye contact as she says this.)
Mrs. Real:	No, dear, I wouldn't mind. But I don't really know it. I think my daughter lives near Hialeah. I'm not sure. My daughter is so careless; she shouldn't have lost me.
Mrs. Tran-Vu:	I'm going to let you rest for a while if that's O.K. with you. Señora Real, how about lunch? Are you interested?

Mrs. Real: Oh, yes, I'd love some lunch. I
               haven't had anything else to eat
               since this morning's breakfast!
               (She smiles.)

Thirty minutes later, Carmen Real, Mrs. Real's daughter, shows up in the emergency department, anxiously looking for her mother. She explains that she had lost her in the mall that morning. She adds that her mother relies on her for her daily activities and does not know or need to know what number to call or how to get back home, thus confirming that her mother was not disoriented.

Using the CARE Approach

Cover the Family. Mrs. Tran-Vu realizes that there may be some family issues involved because the patient is upset with her daughter. Yet, she refrains from encouraging the patient to talk about it. This allows the family's pride to remain intact.

Attention. Mrs. Tran-Vu gives her undivided attention to Mrs. Real. Although at first Mrs. Real resists saying much, Mrs. Tran-Vu's persistent attention and warmth finally win Mrs. Real over.

Respect. Mrs. Tran-vu calls the patient "Señora Real" to show respect. She also records but does not make any judgmental comment regarding Mrs. Real's fear of God.

Eye Contact. While making eye contact, Mrs. Tran-Vu asks questions and encourages the patient to establish a personal connection. Consequently, the patient feels reassured.

Key Points

⇒ Nurse Tran-Vu carries out an initial evaluation of the mental health status of the patient and suspects that there may be cultural issues involved in Mrs. Real's apparent disorientation with respect to time and space. From the conversation, Mrs. Real appears to be strongly dependent on her daughter. Therefore, Mrs. Tran-Vu decides to be supportive and to offer Mrs. Real lunch.

⇒ Although the patient appeared to have a negative attitude, she was, in fact, tired and hungry. Upset and humiliated about finding herself in that situation, she was expecting her daughter to arrive at the hospital at any moment.

Patient 4: Manuel Pérez

This second vignette also highlights strategies to carry out a culturally appropriate mental health evaluation using the CARE approach.

Manuel Pérez is a fifty-five-year-old plumber who emigrated with his wife and two sons from Honduras ten years ago. His wife, a librarian, accompanies him to see Dr. Brown, a clinical psychologist, for the first time.

Dr. Brown: Hello, Señor Pérez, Señora Pérez, I'm Dr. Brown. (He shakes hands and makes eye contact with the patient and his wife.)

Mr. Pérez: I don't really know if I am going to continue seeing you. I was given a referral last week after my wife had to take me to the emergency department (Mr. Pérez says hesitantly).

Mrs. Pérez: I had to drive him to the emergency department; he was too nervous to drive.

Dr. Brown: It seems that the clinician who saw you last week suspects that you are going through some difficult times and may need some help. Have you been taking the medication that he prescribed for you?

Mr. Pérez: No, I decided not to take it. I'm trying to get out of this situation by relaxing. The problem is that bills keep coming in. But I have always been a very responsible father and husband. It's just that with the economic recession, I've had less work, and it really stresses me out. (Dr. Brown notices that Mr. Pérez is on the verge of tears. Mrs. Pérez jumps in.)

Mrs. Pérez: I can attest to that. Manuel has never failed us, never! It's only that this economy is affecting his nerves! He lost his business two months ago; now he's working by himself. I don't understand why God is putting us through this test. (Mr. Pérez starts sobbing.)

Dr. Brown:	I know what you mean. The economy is hitting us all. I even had to sell my house for a price much lower than I had expected.
Mr. Pérez:	My parents are coming to visit from Honduras at the end of the month. I don't want to tell them how bad it is, but my nerves are killing me.
Mrs. Pérez:	We don't have to tell anyone, Manuel. Don't worry. You just have to get treatment for your nerves. At least I still have my job in the library.
Mr. Pérez:	But I've always been the provider of the family!
Dr. Brown:	(Turning to Mr. Pérez, he says,) We're here to help. I know these are tough times, Señor Pérez. You're fortunate to have a wife who supports you all the way. (Turning to Mrs. Pérez he says), We're going to do our best to help you and your family. (He makes deliberate eye contact with Mr. Pérez.)

Using the CARE Approach

Cover the Family. Dr. Brown appreciates the fact that Mr. and Mrs. Pérez have opted to disclose to him their financial tribulations in spite of the fact that most Latinos do not often do so. To reciprocate their trust, he shares with them his own difficulty selling his house.

Attention. At all times, Dr. Brown addresses his remarks to both Mr. and Mrs. Pérez and makes eye contact with both as the conversation progresses, especially when Mr. Pérez is upset.

Respect. Dr. Brown shows respect toward Mr. Pérez' hurt machismo and toward Mrs. Pérez' fear of God's punishment. He addresses both to show respect for their family. At all times, he addresses them respectfully with appropriate titles, "Señor" and "Señora."

Eye Contact. Dr. Brown uses eye contact to convey respect, empathy, attention, and a caring attitude toward the Pérezes.

Key Points

⇒ The Pérezes had been used to a good life until the beginning of the recession. The loss of his business and the impact of this on his role as the provider of the family have sent Mr. Pérez into a spin. Dr. Brown understands that Latino values such as familism, self-worth, machismo, and marianismo are exerting great pressure on Mr. Pérez. Thus, Dr. Brown shows respect toward the couple's Latino values, while at the same time being supportive.

⇒ Dr. Brown uses the CARE approach to establish rapport with Mr. Pérez and his wife. In subsequent interviews he will address Mr. Pérez' particular needs.

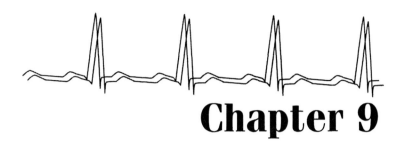

Chapter 9

TREAT: Providing Culturally Competent Treatment

In developing a treatment plan, the level of communication established between the practitioner and the patient will strongly influence the patient's willingness to comply with the provider's therapeutic plan. The family's perception of the provider as a sensitive professional enhances its level of cooperation in helping the patient comply with the suggested treatment plan. The first part of this chapter describes the Latino patient's attitude toward medical as well as health-associated fears. The focus of the second part of the chapter is the TREAT approach, a tool that helps provide culturally competent treatment to Latinos.

Anticipating Patient Reactions to Further Tests

The Latino patient expects the clinician to be able to find the cause of his or her illness and to recommend effective treatment to resolve the problem. The hopes of a patient who seeks help from a health care provider are often high, and in many cases, seeking health care services takes place only after other alternatives have failed. The patient's anxiety and disappointment may increase if, instead of writing a prescription, which is what the patient wants, you request that the patient first undergo tests in order to support the diagnosis. Latino patients meet requests for laboratory or radiographic tests, psychological evaluations, or other diagnostic exams with different reactions.

Laboratory exams are often welcome. Many patients believe that a good provider is careful to make sure that the patient's blood is healthy. Patients sometimes even suggest that a blood test may be needed, reporting that their blood is "thin" (presumed anemia), "thick" (associated with having high cholesterol and high blood pressure), or "hot" (when there is a suspicion of allergies or infections). These health beliefs reflect the hot and cold theory of disease discussed in the first part of this book. From the patient's perspective, urine and stool exams complete the picture that you will need in order to determine how the internal organs are working. Although some elderly patients may express concern about being able to obtain a stool sample promptly due to constipation problems, most patients welcome having their blood, urine, and stools checked.

A request for X rays may suggest to the patient the existence of a more complicated health problem. Still, the patient will probably appreciate your thoroughness. The need for other, more complex radiographic exams, however, may provoke much fearful speculation by the patient and family. For example, an examination of the colon, which requires previous preparation (such as fasting and taking laxatives to clean the intestines prior to the exam), creates anxiety. Generally, the apprehension escalates because the Latino patient interprets the degree of complexity of the exam as an indication of the seriousness of the condition. Therefore, it is of the utmost importance that you explain the reasons for requesting more than the usual number of tests and go over the possible implications of the results with the patient to avoid uneasy speculation by the family. Often, the patient and several family members will be present and will subsequently convey the information to the rest of the family.

The need for a psychological evaluation generally points toward considerable difficulties ahead and can make Latino patients and their families quite anxious. The patient's family members often presume that if psychological or emotional problems are confirmed, the therapy may require a commitment to an undetermined number of appointments. The patient may require special attention that relatives are unable to provide. In addition, complying with appointments with therapists can cause anxiety about job commitments because of the time the adult patient must dedicate to therapy, thus missing work. Worst of all, having a family member undergo treatment for psychological problems can stigmatize some families because of the Latino belief that mental illnesses may reflect problematic family dynamics. No family wants to be labeled as dysfunctional at the community level, especially in the tightly knit Latino community, where word gets around very fast.

Three Considerations Prior to Suggesting a Therapeutic Plan

You may want to explore three issues before prescribing medication or suggesting psychotherapy.

Self-Medication. It is common practice for Latinos to self-medicate. They often save unused medication for future use for symptoms that appear to be similar to those of previous conditions. Relatives, friends, and neighbors may also offer to share their leftover medication, and some readily accept it in hopes of getting better without going through the ordeal of seeking medical attention. Other patients may have access to ethnic community stores where they can buy prescription medication without presenting a provider's prescription.

When asking about self-medication, however, frame the question carefully and avoid projecting a judgmental attitude. For example, you may ask the patient whether any other medications or treatments of any kind have been used to help alleviate the problem prior to the consultation. A patient's positive reply suggests the need to ask the second question.

Folk Healers. Some patients do not report whether they are taking folk medicine as treatment unless you specifically request the information. The best way to ask is to inquire if the patient has seen another doctor in the community. Some patients may give responses such as "Well, I went to see Mr. Ramos last week. He is not a doctor like you, but he's very successful in treating all kinds of problems." Other patients may be wary of disclosing folk practices because of loyalty toward the healer. Healers are very private in their practices, so if a Latino patient is consulting a folk healer, chances are the two may have a long and trusting relationship. After deciding that the provider is trustworthy, patients often share information regarding consultation with their folk healer in subsequent visits to the provider.

A reasonable approach is to inquire about the type of treatment that a folk healer such as Mr. Ramos prescribed in order to determine whether the healer is a curandero(a), a sobador(a), an espiritista, or an herbalist (see pages 62–63). Also determine, if possible, whether the treatment prescribed by the folk healer is harmless to the patient. Unless it is necessary, try to avoid making statements that may be interpreted as critical of or contrary to the folk healer's prescription. If you believe that the patient may be taking a potentially harmful folk medication, one that may be contraindicated or that may interact negatively with prescribed drugs, inform the patient as well as the relatives and offer proper explanations in terms they can clearly understand. Having identified these elements, you may ask the third question.

Drug Presentation Preference. Prescribing a drug in a presentation that the Latino patient prefers will significantly increase compliance with the treatment. Therefore, be sure to ask your patients for their preference. While many will take medication in any presentation, some prefer to take tablets and others favor liquids. Latino patients commonly categorize themselves as "bad tablet takers," "bad syrup takers," "good capsule takers," or "good liquid takers." In some cases, if the presentation of the drug is not to the person's liking, he or she may not even take it.

Finally, in some cases treatment may not be as simple as writing a prescription or suggesting psychotherapy. You may need to indicate the need for other diagnostic procedures or suggest surgery. The negotiation for consent in such cases is often carried out primarily with the Latino patient's family and to a lesser extent with the patient. Therefore, the role of the accompanying relative is monumental, as it involves reporting the outcome of the consultation to other family members, some of whom may even reside in Latin American countries. This family procedure is discussed in the next section.

Negotiating Consent for Diagnostic and Surgical Procedures

As I've just said, giving consent for a diagnostic or surgical procedure is a family affair for most Latinos. Before making a final decision, adults often insist on holding family meetings to seek the advice and opinions of other adult family members, usually brothers, sisters, and even *comadres* ("co-mothers," closest female friends) and *compadres* (male equivalent of comadres). Relatives will appreciate your patience and understanding, especially when the age of the patient is a critical factor in the decision-making process. Adult family members are generally responsible for giving consent to carry out a procedure for a spouse, a child, or an elderly person.

Spouses are protective of their sick partner, and many handle decision-making matters well. They may ask focused questions if they are second or third generation. If they are immigrants, they may seek the advice of relatives or ask a relative to accompany them to help with translation.

Like most parents, Latinos appreciate detailed explanations and are often eager to understand what a procedure involves in terms of its purpose and its risks; yet, because they are so upset and anxious, they may fail to ask focused questions. Their emotional burdens tend to affect their objectivity. In view of this, they may ask brothers, sisters, and cousins to go to the appointment with them and to help with the necessary decisions.

Adult children are traditionally responsible for elderly adults, who tend to voluntarily abdicate responsibility for their own health care and well-being. An elderly Latino or Latina very rarely makes major decisions regarding health issues. If consent is requested for a diagnostic or surgical procedure, elderly Latinos will often tell you that the decision is in the hands of their family. Often, brothers and sisters, children, and even grandchildren convene at an urgent family meeting to discuss the issue, and adults take a vote. If one relative lives out of town or in another country, the meeting (and therefore the procedure) may be postponed for a later date to await the arrival of that person. In other cases, the member who is unable to attend the meeting may delegate the vote to another family member.

After carrying out the diagnostic or surgical procedure, you may want to speak to the head of the family or the closest relative available before you talk with the patient to determine the best way to inform him or her of the outcome. Most patients will appreciate receiving the news if you are accompanied by a family member. In other cases, adult relatives may request that the diagnosis not be disclosed to an elderly patient.

Three Health-Associated Latino Fears

Achieving compliance with treatment and obtaining consent for diagnostic procedures are closely related to the patient's fear of disease, social stigma, and ultimately death. This section presents Latinos' fears associated with health-seeking behaviors.

Fear of Disease

Many Latinos fear illness not only because it affects the family emotionally but also because it has the potential to deplete the family's sometimes meager funds. Because gender roles are clearly defined in the Latino family, the loss of the male provider signifies an almost irreparable financial tragedy. For others, fear of disease may, as I've discussed before, be culturally based; it may be considered a form of punishment from God for bad deeds. In such cases being ill is overwhelming because it is associated with guilt feelings. When explaining the possible causes of an illness to a Latino patient, the provider may want to focus on the physiopathological basis of the disease while emphasizing that in most cases, with proper treatment, the situation may be reversed or improved. Informing a patient and his or her family that the diagnosis is diabetes is a good example. If you explain the causes of the disease while strongly emphasizing the factors that may help the patient lead a normal life, the patient will be more likely to follow the treatment plan. In addition, encouraging the family to ask questions always contributes to increasing their knowledge about the disease and its treatment—and hopefully helps diminish their fears.

Fear of Social Stigma

Although the social family network is often a resource, that same support network may sometimes exert a stigmatizing judgmental attitude. For this reason some families will make an enormous effort to keep secret illnesses that may be considered detrimental to their social standing. For instance, a patient may try to keep a sexually transmitted disease secret, and some families will refrain from disclosing that one of their members has tuberculosis, an infectious disease commonly associated with poverty. Such secrecy may affect the physical or psychological health of others. In the first case, the patient may refuse to locate and inform sexual contacts. In the second case, the family may suffer in silence and make up false stories about the relative's diagnosis.

If the information regarding a patient's illness is transmitted throughout the social or family network, the patient may become the center of negative discussion among such groups, resulting in social stigma for the patient and even the extended family. While chronic diseases are seen with benevolent eyes, some infectious illnesses may trigger moral judgment. Infectious diseases of the respiratory tract in children may be associated with the parents' lack of responsibility for their children. Infectious diseases such as tuberculosis may generate rejection that stems from the fear of being infected. Friends, neighbors, and even relatives may abstain from visiting or being physically close to such a patient, even if the patient is undergoing treatment and is no longer a threat to others. Sexually transmitted diseases can be associated with a moral judgment of the person's sexual behavior.

For all these reasons, when discussing such diseases, special care must be taken to protect the patient's privacy. Asking a relative to leave the office may sometimes be the best approach. In that case, you will be the one to request that the relative leave, because the patient will often refrain from creating friction with a family member. Although your suggestion may not be in tune with Latino collectivism in this case, it is your prerogative to protect the patient's privacy. Family members will accept your request without questioning it out of respect for your authority.

Fear of Death

On one hand Latinos fear death because it implies the loss of a loved one. On the other hand, Catholic Latinos see death as a transition to the afterlife. Either way, death is an unknown zone into which a beloved relative enters, and the unknown creates fear and apprehension for the patient as well as the patient's family. Relatives hope to bravely face the passing away of a relative and to responsibly manage the social and religious duties that their cultural traditions impose on them.

When a patient's condition becomes terminal, relatives have great appreciation for providers who clearly communicate the prognosis to them. This allows Catholic families time to make plans and to manage the situation adequately from a religious perspective. The most critical step for the family is contacting a priest to perform the last rights. This closure is extremely critical to Catholic Latinos. When it is not carried out, relatives are often left feeling remorseful about their deceased relative and resentful toward the provider. When the rite is carried out, relatives feel they have done their duty and feel closer to the provider.

Finally, the family appreciates the respectful treatment of the corpse. Such treatment includes closing the eyelids, covering the body, and maintaining a somber attitude while the deceased is still in the ward. This point is illustrated by Latinos' reaction in the aftermath of the 1988 earthquake in Mexico City. Thousands of relatives angrily resented the insensitive handling of corpses by health authorities and strongly opposed mass graves to dispose of the dead because of the need to celebrate mass and give Christian burial to their deceased family members (Pan American Health Organization 1998).

TREAT: Developing a Culturally Competent Treatment Plan

The TREAT approach helps a provider find the most culturally appropriate manner to establish effective communication with and project sensitivity toward Latinos. The TREAT acronym stands for

T = Touch
R = Respect
E = Empathy
A = Attention
T = Trust

Touch

Touch is a critical element in treating a Latino patient. Placing a hand on the patient's hand while explaining the treatment plan can help the provider communicate more effectively and encourages the patient's compliance with treatment. Showing *and handing a sample of the prescribed medication* to the patient can also establish a symbolic link; you are handing the treatment to the patient and because the patient respects your authority, he or she will be more likely to take the medication.

Respect

Respect is a two-way issue and must be shown by both provider and patient for a treatment plan to succeed. On one hand, you need to show respect to the patient; when your actions convey respect for the patient's cultural health practices, you will often succeed in communicating effectively with the patient and with the patient's family. As I have discussed before, respect for such practices can be demonstrated by refraining from criticizing, being judgmental about, or questioning a treatment suggested by a folk healer. As long as a treatment plan does not conflict with cultural beliefs, most patients will go to great efforts to carry out the plan you suggest. A patient will welcome your suggestion to try a prescribed medication in conjunction with the topical treatment that has been recommended by a folk healer to treat arthritis. At least during the initial visit, it is always best to avoid ruling out the use of herbal remedies that a patient may have been using. If necessary, you can suggest during subsequent visits that the patient stop taking such remedies. In other cases there may be important family implications; some patients use herbal home remedies that may have been recommended by a family member. A grandmother whose herbal medical knowledge is highly respected may have recommended the use of tea infusions. Asking the pa-

tient to discontinue their use may create a conflict
between either the patient and the relative or you and
the patient. Thus, it is best to avoid interfering with
family matters if the home remedy does not appear to
interfere with the treatment or is innocuous. Another
key element of showing respect toward a patient is
the use of appropriate titles to address the patient. Informally addressing patients by their first names is often not welcome, especially by immigrants.

On the other hand, the patient's respect for the
provider is equally important if a treatment plan is to
succeed. Most patients have a respectful attitude toward providers because they assume that clinical
knowledge gives them the power to cure. When Latino
patients seek care, they hope for full recovery and often comment that they "will place themselves in their
doctor's hands"; and families say they "have faith in
the provider." Other patients have a different kind of
respect toward the clinician. They often comment they
have faith in the provider because "God is guiding the
doctor's hands and mind." The family's respect is often
earned after one family member's successful recovery.
Subsequently, the rest of the family will attest to the
clinician's scientific knowledge and will often recommend the practitioner to relatives and friends. Thus, it
is not unlikely for a provider to be chosen by all the
members of the same family.

You may want to ask relatives if an elderly patient
is to be informed of the diagnosis and treatment plan
before discussing it with the patient. In some cases, as
I've said elsewhere, family members withhold this in-

formation from elderly patients. Failure to reveal the actual health condition to such a patient should not be judged as inappropriate, because it is part of Latinos' paternalistic attitude toward their elderly. They intend to spare the elderly family member suffering if the condition is progressive or if there are slim chances of recovery with treatment.

Empathy

Compassion and understanding are critical elements in negotiating a treatment plan with the patient and the patient's family. Patients tend to be very sensitive to your tone of voice and facial expression. At times, a warm smile will add a great deal of empathy to the interaction. A smile may convey your down-to-earth attitude and will help ameliorate the power differential between patient and provider. Family members are usually protective of their sick, a fact that helps ensure compliance with prescribed treatments. For this reason, being culturally aware, showing support, and maintaining a reassuring attitude will help you establish a relationship with the patient and the patient's family that is conducive to compliance (Delgado 1998).

Attention

Your full attention is essential when you are recommending psychotherapy or prescribing medication. In both cases your attentiveness will encourage compliance. If you can reiterate an interest in the patient's well-being and combine such a statement with eye contact, you will inspire compliance. Eye contact with the patient is important even if the patient has limited English proficiency and you are working with an interpreter. Address all of your remarks to the patient, not the interpreter. Many Latino patients evaluate a provider on the basis of the degree of attention they perceive from the clinician. Unsatisfied Latino patients' common complaint is, "The doctor didn't even pay attention to me."

When recommending psychotherapy, attention to the accompanying family members is also essential because they can be your allies. In many cases, the family's participation is needed in the period following a patient's hospital discharge. When relatives perceive that you care about the patient and respect the family's health beliefs, they will often return to seek your help and support in caring for the patient and for other family members.

Latinos expect to walk out of your office with a prescription in their hand; they interpret this prescription as a symbol of your attention to their well-being. In fact, the prescription is high on the list of criteria that Latinos use to informally evaluate a provider; it is perceived as a reflection of the extent to which the provider understands the patient's needs. When there is no need to prescribe a medication, suggesting that patients take vitamins is always received with enthusiasm because they interpret the recommendation as proof of your direct and personal interest in keeping them healthy. Latinos believe that working long hours takes a toll on the body and requires vitamins to "reconstitute" it. In fact, they call vitamins and similar over-the-counter products *reconstituyentes*. They believe that vitamins will help them regain stamina.

Trust

Most Latino patients are looking for a provider who will be trustworthy and interested in improving their health status. The two best ways to gain their trust are to avoid being judgmental toward their beliefs and practices and to relate to them on a personal level. On using herbal remedies, you may comment, "I take herbal teas myself sometimes." Also demonstrate personalismo by relating to the Latino patient and family on a personal basis. One way of making this personal connection is to ask them to share family recipes and experiences pertaining to recent visits to their countries of origin. Making a comment such as "I was in…two years ago and would like to go back next year" may help display personalismo.

TREAT in Practice

The TREAT approach is a useful tool to assist the clinician in gaining the Latino patient's respect and trust through touch, empathy, and attention. TREAT increases the likelihood of the patient's cooperation and helps ensure family support for the suggested disease management plan. The next two vignettes illustrate the use of the TREAT approach by two providers.

Patient 1: Nelly Huertas

Mrs. Nelly Huertas is a fifty-nine-year-old Latina who

immigrated to the United States in 1960. Every year she returns to Mexico on vacation to visit her relatives and friends. After she returned from the trip last year, she developed a persistent cough, lost nearly twenty pounds, and eventually found out she had tuberculosis. She goes to her appointment with Mrs. Scott, the nurse in charge of her case at the outpatient clinic. This is Nelly Huertas' sixth appointment with Mrs. Scott.

Mrs. Scott:	Hi, Señora Huertas. How are you feeling today?
Mrs. Huertas:	Well, not so great. The cough is driving me crazy. It's embarrassing sometimes. I don't seem to be gaining much weight, either. Some neighbors have started making comments about my cough. The other day somebody was joking and said my cough sounds like tuberculosis. I thought I was going to die of humiliation that day. If they found out that I really do have tuberculosis, they would probably think I got sick in Mexico, and they would imagine that my family there is living in poverty.
Mrs. Scott:	I understand what you mean. (Mrs. Scott's tone of voice is reassuring.) I had an uncle who had tuberculosis years ago. My family also worried a lot about

him. I even took care of him while
I was in nursing school. Well, I
have great news. You gained two
pounds over the last month, and
your chest X ray looks much
better. Have you been taking your
medication as prescribed?

Mrs. Huertas: Yes, but I feel bad about my
husband. I try to stay away from
him because I don't want him to
get sick. He tells me that he loves
me and that all he wants is for me
to be healthy.

Mrs. Scott: I'm glad he's supportive of you. But
you know you need not be con-
cerned about infecting him,
because you are taking medication. (Mrs. Scott places her hand
on Mrs. Huertas' hand.)

Mrs. Huertas: Yes, I can't complain about him.
But some of my relatives have
stopped visiting us. They used to
come to our house every week
until they found out I have this
awful disease. Sometimes I don't
even feel like taking the medication. (Mrs. Scott listens attentively
and with an empathetic expression
of concern.)

Mrs. Scott: The treatment seems to be working very well. I understand it must
be very difficult for you. Does

	your husband understand what you are going through?
Mrs. Huertas:	Yes, he does. He's very helpful and tells me I shouldn't worry about my relatives. But it's very hard to be rejected by my own family. Do you know what I mean?
Mrs. Scott:	Yes, I do, Señora Huertas. We must make sure that you get well as soon as possible; that is our main concern. As soon as you regain your health, things will start to get better, don't you think?
Mrs. Huertas:	I sure hope so. But it hurts a lot to think that my relatives are talking about me all the time. I hate them sometimes.
Mrs. Scott:	Señora Huertas, do you think it might help you to talk to a psychologist and maybe get those feelings out? We have a very good psychologist here.
Mrs. Huertas:	Yes, Mrs. Scott. I think it might help.

Using the TREAT Approach

Touch. Mrs. Scott has extensive experience working with Latinos. She understands that Mrs. Huertas needs to talk about her social and family life more than about her disease. While Mrs. Huertas is talking, Mrs. Scott places her hand on the patient's hand.

Respect. Mrs. Scott shows respect in several ways. First, she calls the patient by her last name preceded by the title, "Señora." Second, she shows that she understands the role of Mrs. Huertas' husband in her life as well as the importance of her relatives. Mrs. Scott knows that Latinos fear tuberculosis because they perceive it as a highly infectious disease that therefore may affect the social life of the family.

Empathy. Mrs. Scott conveys empathy by using a tone of voice that is very mellow and reassuring and by presenting a very concerned but hopeful expression on her face. Although the patient is complying with the treatment and it seems to be working, she appears to be in need of psychological support in addition to her husband's moral support.

Attention. Mrs. Scott listens attentively and understands the importance of the social support network among Latinos. She suggests an appointment with a psychologist to help Mrs. Huertas cope with the social rejection she is experiencing.

Trust. Telling Mrs. Huertas about her own family's experience with a relative who contracted tuberculosis helps Mrs. Scott relate to Mrs. Huertas on a personal level. It reveals Mrs. Scott's personalismo to the patient.

Key Points

⇒ Mrs. Scott makes efforts to prevent the patient from getting discouraged by social pressures because it could interfere with her compliance with the prescribed treatment.

⇒ Mrs. Huertas' condition appears to be improving and, with psychological support and a respectful attitude toward her, she should continue to adhere to the prescribed treatment.

Patient 2: Roberto Torres

Roberto Torres is an overweight, elderly Nicaraguan immigrant. He is seventy-five years old and is accompanied by his daughter, Marta Torres, a single, thirty-five-year-old bilingual woman who works as an assistant manager in a department store. When they walk in the office, Dr. Jones, Mr. Torres' primary care physician for the last year, shakes hands with the patient first and then his daughter. Mr. Torres speaks little English, so Dr. Jones must rely on his daughter to act as interpreter.

Dr. Jones: Hello, Señor Torres. I last saw you two months ago. We have all the results of your tests here in your file. (Dr. Jones makes eye contact with Mr. Torres as he speaks. He then turns to Miss Torres, who has just translated his words for her father.)

Dr. Jones: Hello, Miss Torres. How are you?

Miss Torres: I'm very worried about my father. If there is anything wrong with his health, I need to know. But I'd like to ask you to please not tell him if there's anything seriously wrong because my brothers and sisters would prefer not to tell him. He's too old, you know? We just want

	him to have a good life during his last years.
Dr. Jones:	Yes. Of course. Let's talk about the laboratory results first. (He turns back to Mr. Torres.)
Dr. Jones:	Señor Torres, your hemoglobin count is fine. That's good news. We may have to refer you to the nutritionist, though. The fat in your diet may not be helping your health. (Miss Torres continues to translate.)
Mr. Torres:	O.K. (He moves his head affirmatively.)
Dr. Jones:	Do you exercise often? (Dr. Jones asks this with a friendly smile.)
Mr. Torres:	Yes. (He nods his head affirmatively and laughs.)
Miss Torres:	He moves his arms and legs when he's watching television. He says that's his exercise.
Dr. Jones:	Well, is there a possibility that you can take a short walk every day, Señor Torres?
Miss Torres:	He would like to walk around the block, but at home we all work so there's nobody to go with him. I don't like him to go out by himself anymore. He fell one time and hit his head on the curb. Thank God nothing bad happened.
Dr. Jones:	O.K., let me see. Señor Torres, if

	your family could find a neighbor to walk with you every morning, would you like to do it?
Mr. Torres:	(He moves his head affirmatively, smiling.)
Miss Torres:	I guess that's something that we could do. We have two neighbors who would probably be willing to walk with father. It's his heart, right, Dr. Jones?
Dr. Jones:	Probably, Miss Torres. I believe his coronary arteries may be partially obstructed. We will need to have him go through some other tests that will allow us to get a pretty accurate picture of his arteries. It will be very helpful to have this information so we can decide what to do next to help your father.
Dr. Jones:	Señor Torres, We're going to take good care of you. (He makes eye contact and smiles at his patient.)
Mr. Torres:	O.K.
Miss Torres:	Is there risk in the tests, Dr. Jones? I need to report this to my brothers and sisters. I have a sister who lives in Nicaragua. Do you think she should come?
Dr. Jones:	Well, Miss Torres, that's a decision that your family may want to discuss. However, his condition appears to be stable right now.

Dr. Jones:	(He turns to Mr. Torres.) Have you had any more chest pains since your last visit?
Mr. Torres:	(He shakes his head negatively.)
Dr. Jones:	I'm going to prescribe some medication for you. Are you good with tablets or do you prefer liquid medication? (He says this as he places his hand on the patient's.)
Miss Torres:	He says he prefers liquid medication. He's a terrible tablet taker. He also wants to know if he can continue taking an herbal tea that Maestro Guzmán prescribed for him when he was feeling tired. It's chamomile tea.
Dr. Jones:	Yes, that's fine; please tell him to keep taking the tea in addition to what I'm prescribing. (turning to face Mr. Torres) Here's the prescription. (He hands it to Mr. Torres, who immediately gives it to his daughter.)
Miss Torres:	May I call you later to talk about his condition?
Dr. Jones:	Yes, please do. Here's my card. I often have some time to talk in the late afternoon. You can have me paged in the hospital. (He turns to Mr. Torres and smiles.)
Dr. Jones:	Señor Torres, I'm going to give you a referral to the nutritionist and I'm going to indicate some more tests.

> After I see the results of the tests, I may recommend that you try to take a short walk in the mornings. Please don't forget to take your tea and the medication, O.K.? I would like to see you again in a month. (Dr. Jones speaks to the patient while shaking his hand.) Please say hello to the family, O.K.?

Mr. Torres: Yes, thank you.

Using the TREAT Approach

Touch. When the patient enters his office, Dr. Jones shakes hands with Mr. Torres first and then with Miss Torres to acknowledge her presence. Throughout the interview, Dr. Jones puts his hand on Mr. Torres' hand often. Mr. Torres is an elderly person; therefore, the gesture is appropriate. Mr. Torres most likely appreciates it.

Respect. Throughout the consultation, Dr. Jones addresses the patient as "Señor Torres" and his single daughter as "Miss Torres" to show respect to both. Although the patient speaks little English, Dr. Jones addresses him and makes eye contact with him frequently while his daughter acts as interpreter. Dr. Jones prescribes a medication and suggests that Mr. Torres take it in addition to his herbal tea, showing respect for the patient's health practices. Maestro Guzmán is the family folk healer.

Empathy. Dr. Jones smiles often while explaining the treatment plan to make sure that the patient feels cared for. At the end of the interview, he sends a greeting to the family. Dr. Jones understands that Miss Torres is responsible for her father and that she must report to the family. He respects the family's possible decision to not disclose the severity of the illness to the patient.

Attention. Dr. Jones explains the treatment to the patient and understands that the patient will not ask questions because he relies on his daughter to take care of this matter. He makes frequent eye contact with the patient and his daughter, ensuring that they understand that they have his undivided attention.

Trust. Dr. Jones is not judgmental toward Mr. Torres' health practices (using tea) and relates to his patient and his patient's daughter on a personal level, with open personalismo, friendliness, and approachability. He gives his business card to Mr. Torres' daughter so that she can call him later to talk about her father's health.

Key Points

⇒ Dr. Jones displays cultural sensitivity toward his Latino patient. He understands that family dynamics are very important in supporting the patient's compliance with the treatment. Dr. Jones will communicate the details of the additional tests and the therapeutic plan to the patient's daughter later, by phone.

⇒ When explaining that he will request additional tests, Dr. Jones offers a brief explanation to Miss Torres in order to share with her what he has in mind.

⇒ Understanding that the family will be involved in the decision to carry out additional tests, he provides an open opinion regarding the possibility of contacting Miss Torres' sister, who does not live in the United States.

⇒ Fear of disease and fear of death are in Miss Torres' mind. Knowing this, Dr. Jones makes special efforts to provide clear explanations that may dispel some of her fears. Mr. Torres does not exhibit any fear because he is not informed of his condition.

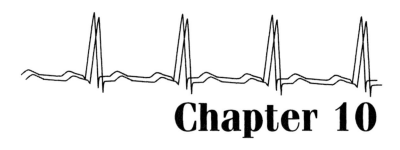

Chapter 10

Developing Patient Loyalty and the Effective Farewell

The diversity of the Latino population presents a formidable challenge to health care providers. While there are shared cultural values in the group, critical social and demographic issues set them apart. In addition each patient is an individual and is therefore unique. To help overcome some of these obstacles, this book has attempted to highlight, describe, and explain the cultural values that are most commonly shared by Latinos and that emerge in the patient-provider encounter. Just as the Spanish language unites all Latinos, loyalty is characteristic of many Latino patients. The majority yearn to find a health provider whom they can connect with and respect in order to establish a lasting patient-provider relationship.

What Is Patient Loyalty?

Advertising agencies often describe Latinos as a loyal market because they usually maintain their preferences long after making initial choices regarding products and services (Fisher 1994; Albonetti and Dominguez 1989). Advertisers also keenly observe demographic trends. Knowing that 35 percent of the U.S. Hispanic population is under the age of eighteen, they have begun to cultivate that market to create brand loyalty among future Latino adults (Giegoldt 1998; Ebenkamp and Khermouch 1996). The concept of Latino loyalty also extends to Latinos' behavior toward health care providers. However, there are circumstances that complicate the situation.

First, working in lower-paid jobs often stands in the way of Latinos' access to health care services. In fact, Latinos account for 35 percent of the nation's uninsured population. Second, the health care needs of Latinos are not fully documented because there is still not enough data available. Third is the need to provide culturally and linguistically appropriate services to Latinos. Having health insurance is a priority for most Latinos despite a system that may not be fully prepared to respond to their needs, and the fact that they must circumvent obstacles to have access to health services makes them appreciate these services even more. Once in the system, Latinos actively seek the right provider, and when they find that person, the link is often maintained for many years. The definition of loyalty toward the provider comes in many shapes and forms, as is illustrated in the following three examples.

Tomás and María Puente

Tomás and María Puente moved from Puerto Rico to New York City ten years ago. Since that time they have taken their three children to only two health clinics. Ricky, their youngest son, is asthmatic. Dr. Tom Neal has known Ricky since he was born; he even knows when the boy may be more prone to an asthmatic attack because he understands the boy. Two years ago Tomás and María sought services at another clinic in order to follow Dr. Neal, who had changed jobs. He is the provider they trust. Tomás and María consider Dr. Neal a friend of the family and share with him the family's private and public successes and defeats. They will follow Dr. Neal if he goes to work in another facility, no matter how far. For the Puente family, loyalty means giving back the caring attitude they receive from Dr. Neal, who knows and understands their trials and tribulations. Dr. Neal is a trusted friend and family doctor.

Josefina González

A seventy-year-old immigrant from Mexico, Josefina González is sure that she owes her life to Dr. Jane Owens. Mrs. González immigrated to the United

States twenty years ago, along with her husband José and their two children. After her husband passed away, she moved in with her married daughter Maria and her family. María has been looking after her for the past ten years. Mrs. González met Dr. Owens five years ago when she required urgent medical attention after she passed out at home. Dr. Owens diagnosed Mrs. González with diabetes and hypertension. Mrs. González believes that Dr. Owens saved her life because she diagnosed two illnesses that would have gone undetected had she not gone to the hospital that night. Mrs. González reports that she is in Dr. Owens' hands and will do anything that Dr. Owens suggests. For example, she reports, "Dr. Owens prohibited that I eat sweets and I don't. If it weren't for Dr. Owens, I would be blind and I probably wouldn't be able to walk by now." Mrs. González has faith in Dr. Owens' clinical abilities because she is always very accurate in prescribing medication that keeps her healthy. Faith and trust are the expressions of her loyalty.

Roberto Lopez

Roberto Lopez is a college-educated Cuban American who works as a top-level executive in Miami. He is fifty-five years old, married, and has two sons in college. Roberto was referred to Dr. John Lowe, a clinical psychologist, five years ago because he was experiencing sexual dysfunction. Dr. Lowe helped Roberto deal with his stress and anxiety at work and at home. Although Dr. Lowe has changed jobs twice since Roberto first went to see him, Roberto has followed him. Having shared with Dr. Lowe his most private and personal fears and problems, Roberto feels he has a friend in Dr. Lowe. Twice a year he requests an appointment with Dr. Lowe only to touch base; his insecurities are not a major problem now. For Roberto loyalty is a result of having shared private information, of having had positive results with the provider, and of having developed a trusting relationship with him over the years.

In these three examples, the Puentes believe that the provider cares about their health, Josefina González believes her provider saved their life, and Roberto Lopez trusts his provider with very private personal information. Each patient has a personal definition of loyalty. Yet the three cases suggest a number of common characteristics. The next section describes four elements that help define a caring provider from the Latino perspective.

A Caring Provider: The Patient's Perspective

Latinos have a Spanish word to describe a caring health provider, *cariñoso*. A cariñoso clinician is one who shows affection toward the patient, which, by the way, need not be a show of emotion. *Cariñoso* implies that the patient was satisfied with the delivery of services because he or she perceived a personal touch in the provider-patient relationship. Latino patient satisfaction comes from four elements of the encounter: the time the provider spends with the patient, the type of attention the patient perceives, the degree of comfort the patient feels during the encounter, and the assurance that the provider is interested in the well-being of the patient.

Time Spent with the Patient

As mentioned in earlier chapters, Latinos are very relaxed about time. In contrast, the mainstream culture values time as a commodity. Built into the current health care system are time constraints that limit the amount of time that a provider can spend with a patient. Latinos know this; however, it appears that they do not resent time restrictions as much as they do a mainstream provider who is objective and to the point but who makes no attempt to form a personal connection with them. There are at least two ways to be objective and to the point while also being sensitive to personalismo and other aspects of Latino culture.

Leave the door open for a future consultation. A patient seeking a consultation believes that he or she has a real health problem. Often, simply talking about the problem helps alleviate the symptoms. At other times Latinos go to a provider to talk about their concerns regarding several subjects. A mother, for example, may be worried and anxious about her teenage daughter getting pregnant or about her son getting hooked on drugs as well as her own health complaint. She will be very upset and disappointed if you simply tell her that there is nothing wrong and then dismiss her. Instead, listen to her concerns, offer suggestions or a referral, then suggest that the patient return if the problem occurs again. Managing the encounter in a way that leaves a welcoming door open for a future consultation is important for Latinos for two reasons. First, patients feel reassured that the provider is not trying to get them out the door. Second, it conveys to the patient that the provider believes in the existence of the patient's illness and problems.

Guide the patient. When possible, guide the patient to talk about signs and symptoms, instead of asking direct questions. Latino patients interpret direct questions as a desire to end the visit. Guiding a patient is a matter of courteously interrupting whenever the patient begins to roam onto other subjects. For example, instead of asking questions in order to keep the patient's description of the illness focused, try to make comments that encourage the patient to elaborate on specific issues. The following guiding comments and their effects may be helpful.

⇒ "It seems like you've had this problem for a long time."

   Generally, this comment triggers a narration of
   the problem, from its beginning to the current
   status.

⇒ "So the pain didn't allow you to get up and go to work."

   The patient will go into great detail to describe
   the type of pain and whether it was incapaci-
   tating enough to prevent him or her from
   going to work or engaging in other activities.

⇒ "Many families have this illness."

Hearing this comment makes the patient able to relax and discuss the presence or absence of the disease in the family.

⇒ "Some people get sick when they do that."
The comment helps determine if the habit the patient is discussing has been the source of previous illnesses. It also puts the patient at ease instead of feeling that he or she has a unique problem.

⇒ "Gaining weight is so easy."
Making this comment to an overweight patient projects an understanding attitude. By not feeling that the provider is judgmental, the patient often reacts positively to the need to lose weight.

Type of Attention the Patient Perceives

In contrast with mainstream patients who are often more focused on getting treatment, Latinos who seek health care services have high expectations of the attention they will receive. They look forward to having the undivided, personal attention of the provider. When this happens, they often comment that the provider was *atento*, or attentive. There are four ways to project attentiveness, all of which have been discussed in previous chapters:

1. Listen actively by making short, one-syllable comments such as "oh," "ah," "so," and "mmm."
2. Make eye contact as often as possible and appropriate to confirm to the patient that you are engaged in the conversation.

3. Do not allow unnecessary interruptions from staff members; the patient often perceives these as a lack of respect.
4. Show a friendly attitude and share personal experiences. This tells the patient that you are paying attention and that you understand what the patient is saying because you've also experienced it.

Degree of Comfort the Patient Feels

When patients feel at ease, they often give valuable information to the provider. Latinos describe feeling at ease as having *confianza*. This term implies that the patient perceives a sufficient degree of closeness with the clinician to allow the disclosure of private and personal information. In other words, the patient trusts the provider. Three ways to help a patient develop confianza are as follows:

1. Use facial expressions to show concern about the patient's health problem.
2. Avoid reacting in any way that may be perceived by the patient as judgmental.
3. Explicitly express interest in helping improve the patient's health.

The Provider's Interest in the Patient's Well-Being

Latino patients have a pressing need to feel cared for by the provider. In most cases the provider may ask at the end of the visit if the patient is taking vitamins. Latinos interpret the question as a provider's direct and personal interest in keeping the patient healthy. By

suggesting that a patient take vitamins and even discussing the type of vitamins, you are telling the patient, "I want you to stay healthy for me."

A Caring Provider:
The Provider's Perspective

A working definition of the "caring provider" would
be one who understands personalismo and practices
simpatía. In so doing, the provider develops patient
loyalty. Both personalismo and simpatía have been discussed at length in chapter 2 and mentioned throughout the book. I summarize here only.

Understanding Personalismo

The need for Latinos to perceive a personal touch in
the clinical encounter cannot be emphasized enough.
The mainstream health care culture often places a great
deal of weight on professional image. In contrast,
Latino patients seek a friendly person willing to listen
and offer help in solving perceived health problems.
A friendly provider is said to have a great deal of
personalismo. It is a positive trait that encourages communication with Latinos and in return usually generates a great deal of respect for the provider.

Practicing Simpatía

Simpatía, the development of a harmonious relationship with the patient and the patient's family, is
achieved by showing a warm and caring attitude. A
provider described as simpático does not create con-

flict with the patient or with the family; the interaction is very smooth. Patient and family regard the provider as a dear friend whom they can turn to when they need help.

In sum, the key to success with a Latino patient is to establish personal interaction and maintain a harmonious encounter in addition to using GREET during the initial encounter, LISTEN to carry out the interview, CARE to examine the patient, and TREAT to negotiate a therapeutic plan. In this way you establish a cordial relationship with the Latino patient and the patient's family. Delivering good quality care (from the Latino perspective) lays the foundation for a strong professional and personal tie that can result in patient loyalty, as reflected in patient retention rates.

There is one final step. The way in which a provider brings the appointment to an end seals the patient-provider relationship. The farewell is as important as expressing personalismo and simpatía.

The Effective Farewell Pyramid

The effective farewell process begins the moment the provider has fulfilled all the steps of the encounter and the patient gets ready to leave the provider's office. To make a lasting impression on a Latino patient and family and show them respect, consider the six steps in the farewell pyramid:

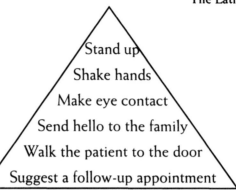

Stand up
Shake hands
Make eye contact
Send hello to the family
Walk the patient to the door
Suggest a follow-up appointment

Stand up. Out of respect for your professional position, the patient will seldom stand up first. Therefore, when you stand up, the patient gets the message that the consultation has ended.

Shake hands. Latinos always appreciate a handshake because they are members of a contact culture. Holding a patient's hands between both of your hands can transmit an even warmer message and is appropriate, if done briefly.

Make eye contact. Making eye contact, smiling, and shaking hands go together and add a personal touch to the farewell process. These acts are personalismo in action.

Send hello to the family. Even if you have not met the rest of the family, sending them a greeting implies a desire to maintain cordial and harmonious relations with the patient and the patient's family. If family members are present, smile, shake hands, and make eye contact with each person.

Walk the patient to the door. Leading a patient toward the door is a welcome gesture, and it also helps you control time. Patients perceive being accompanied to the door as a sign of respect.

Suggest a follow-up appointment. When you suggest a follow-up appointment, the patient feels that you have taken a personal interest in the case, and you feel that adequate communication and rapport were established with the patient. Offering a business card to a patient or relative can create an even more lasting impression. It conveys the message, "I am here whenever you need me." Most Latino patients will not use the card, but they will keep it in a safe place at home; it will give them a sense of security.

*   *   *   *   *   *

As promised in the Introduction of this book, in Part I, I presented Latino cultural beliefs and practices as well as the health status of this population and the concept of cultural competence as it applies to Latinos. In Part II, I presented culturally appropriate approaches and illustrative vignettes that you may find useful during the clinical encounter with Latino patients. Emphasis was placed on sharing a variety of alternatives from which you may choose, depending on your personal style. The Latino culture in the United States is still evolving as new generations of Latinos appear. Therefore, the project remains a work in progress.

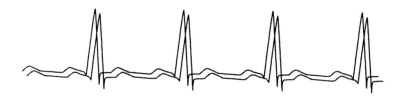

Bibliography

Abraido-Lanza, Ana F., Bruce P. Dohrenwend, Daisy S. Ng-Mak, and J. Blake Turner. 1999. "The Latino Mortality Paradox: A Test of the 'Salmon Bias' and Healthy Migrant Hypotheses." *American Journal of Public Health* 89, no. 10: 1543–51.

Ailinger, Rita L., and Margaret R. Dear. 1997. "Latino Immigrants' Explanatory Models of Tuberculosis." *Qualitative Health Research* 7, no. 4: 521–31.

Albonetti, Joseph G., and Luis V. Dominguez. 1989. "Major Influences on Consumer-Goods Marketers' Decision to Target U.S. Hispanics." *Journal of Advertising Research* 29, no. 1: 9–22.

Alcalay, Rina, Matilda Alvarado, Hector Balcazar, Eileen Newman, and Elmer Huerta. 1999. "Salud para su corazón: A Community-based Latino Cardiovascular Disease Prevention and Outreach Model." *Journal of Community Health* 24, no. 5: 359–79.

Alcalay, Rina, Annette Ghee, and Susan Scrimshaw. 1993.
    "Designing Prenatal Care Messages for Low-Income
    Mexican Women." *Public Health Reports* 108, no. 3:
    354–62.

Alcalay, Rina, Fabio Sabogal, and Joanne R. Gribble. 1992.
    "Profile of Latino Health and Implications for
    Health Education." *International Quarterly of Community Health Education* 12, no. 2: 151–62.

American Medical Association. 1999. *Cultural Competence Compendium*, 2d ed.

American Psychological Association. 2000. *Guidelines for Providers of Psychological Services to Ethnic, Linguistic, and Culturally Diverse Populations.* www.apa.org/pi/
    publicat.html#oema

Axtell, Roger E. 1991. *Gestures: The Dos and Taboos of Body Language around the World.* New York: John Wiley and
    Sons.

Baezconde-Garbanati, Lourdes, Carmen Portillo, and James
    A. Garbanati. 1999. "Disparities in Health Indicators for Latinas in California." *Hispanic Journal of Behavioral Sciences* 21, no. 3: 302–304.

Balcazar, Hector, Felipe G. Castro, and Jennifer L. Krull.
    1995. "Cancer Risk Reduction in Mexican American Women: The Role of Acculturation, Education,
    and Health Risk Factors." *Health Education Quarterly* 22, no. 1: 61–84.

Balcazar, Hector, Gary W. Peterson, and Jennifer L. Krull.
    1997. "Acculturation and Family Cohesiveness in
    Mexican American Pregnant Women: Social and
    Health Implications." *Family and Community Health* 20,
    no. 3: 16–31.

Bell, Robert A., and Rina Alcalay. 1997. "The Impact of the
    Wellness Guide-Guia on Hispanic Women's Well-

being-related Knowledge, Efficacy Beliefs, and Behaviors: The Mediating Role of Acculturation."
Health Education and Behavior 24, no. 3: 326–43.

Bennett, Milton. J. 1993. "Towards Ethnorelativism: A De-
velopmental Model of Intercultural Sensitivity." In
Education for the Intercultural Experience, edited by R.
Michael Paige. Yarmouth, ME: Intercultural Press.

Berk, Mark L., Claudia L. Schur, Leo R. Chavez, and Mar-
tin Frankel. 2000. "Health Care Use among Undocumented Latino Immigrants." *Health Affairs* 19,
no. 4: 51–64.

Black, Sandra A., and Kyriakos S. Markides. 1993. "Acculturation and Alcohol Consumption in Puerto Rican,
Cuban-American, and Mexican American Women
in the United States." *American Journal of Public Health*
83, no. 6: 890–93.

Bureau of the Census. 2001. Population Projections Program, Projections of the Resident Population by
Race, Hispanic Origin, and Nativity: Middle Series, 2050–2070. NP-T5-G.

Bureau of the Census. 2000. National Vital Statistics Reports 48, no. 11: 37.

Bureau of the Census. 2000. Census Bureau Facts for Fea-
tures, CB00-FF.11, 11 September.

Bureau of the Census. 1999. Census Bureau Facts for Fea-
tures, CB99-FF12, 13 September.

Bureau of the Census. 1993. "The Hispanic Population in
the United States: March 1993." *Current Population
Reports*, Population Characteristics Series P20-475.

Bureau of the Census. 1993. *We the American Hispanics*. Washington, DC: United States Government Printing
Office.

Caetaño, Raul, and Maria Elena M. Mora. 1988. "Acculturation and Drinking among People of Mexican Descent in Mexico and the United States." *Journal of Studies on Alcohol* 49, no. 5: 462–71.

Campinha-Bacote, Josepha. 1994. *The Process of Cultural Competence in Health Care: A Culturally Competent Model of Care.* 2d ed. Cincinnati, OH: Transcultural C.A.R.E.

Carrasquillo, Olveen, Angeles I. Carrasquillo, and Stephen Shea. 2000. "Health Insurance Coverage of Immigrants Living in the United States: Differences by Citizenship Status and Country of Origin." *American Journal of Public Health* 90, no. 6: 917–28.

Casas, Juan M., Alfredo Bimbela, Carla V. Corral, Isidro Yañez, Randall C. Swaim, Jeffrey C. Wayman, and Scott Bates. 1998. "Cigarette and Smokeless Tobacco Use among Migrant and Nonmigrant Mexican American Youth." *Hispanic Journal of Behavioral Sciences* 20, no. 1: 102–21.

Centro San Bonifacio. 1997. *Nuestra Cultura, Nuestra Salud: A Handbook on Latin American Health Beliefs and Practices.* The Robert Wood Johnson Foundation and The Henry J. Kaiser Family Foundation.

Cervantes, Richard C., M. Jean Gilbert, Nelly Salgado de Snyder, and Amado Padilla. 1991. "Psychosocial Correlates of Alcohol Use in Younger Adult Immigrant and U.S.-born Hispanics." *The International Journal of the Addictions* 25, no. 5A-6A: 687–708.

Chase, Robert, and Clarisa M. Chase. 1998. *An Introduction to Spanish for Health Care Workers.* New Haven, CT: Yale University Press.

Cohen, Elena, and Tawara D. Goode. 1999. *Policy Brief 1: Rationale for Cultural Competence in Primary Care.* Washington, DC: National Center for Cultural Competence.

Council on Scientific Affairs. 1991. "Hispanic Health in the United States." *Journal of the American Medical Association* 265: 248–52.

Cross, Terry L., Barbara J. Bazron, Karl W. Dennis, and Mareasa R. Isaacs. 1989. *Towards a Culturally Competent System of Care: Vol. 1.* Washington, DC: National Technical Assistance Center for Children's Mental Health, Georgetown University Child Development Center.

Davis, Sharon, and Virginia Chavez. 1995. "Hispanic Households." In *Hispanic Psychology*, edited by Amado Padilla. Thousand Oaks, CA: Sage Publications.

Delgado, Jane L. 1998. "Meeting the Health Promotion Needs of Hispanic Communities." *American Journal of Health Promotion* 9, no. 4: 300–310.

Delgado, Jane L., and Leobardo Estrada. 1993. "Improving Data Collection Strategies." *Public Health Reports* 108, no. 5: 540–46.

Ebenkamp, Becky, and Gerry Khermouch. 1996. "Why Major Marketers are Latin Lovers." *Brandweek* 37, no. 32: 20–24.

Fisher, Christy. 1994. "Hispanic Media See Siesta Ending; Entrance of Big-Name Marketers Leads to 14% Ad Revenue Jump." *Advertising Age* 65, no. 4: S1–2.

Furiño, Antonio, and Eric Muñoz. 1991. "Health Status among Hispanics: Major Themes and New Priorities." *Journal of the American Medical Association* 265, no. 2: 255–57.

Gardiner, Clinton H. 1975. *The Japanese and Peru, 1873–1973.* Albuquerque: University of New Mexico Press.

Gelfand, Donald E. 1989. "Immigration, Aging and Intergenerational Relationships." *Gerontologist* 29, no. 3: 366–73.

General Accounting Office. 1992. "Hispanic Access to Health Care: Significant Gaps Exist." United States General Accounting Office, Report to Congressional Requesters, GAO/PEMD-92-6.

Giegoldt, Laura. 1998. "Brand Loyalty Opportunities Abound: As Teen Market Grows, so Does Challenge to Reach Bilingual Niche." *Advertising Age* 69, no. 34: 58.

Gil, Rosa M., and Carmen I. Vazquez. 1996. *The Maria Paradox.* New York: The Berkley Publishing Group.

Gilbert, M. Jean. 1991. "Acculturation and Changes in Drinking Patterns among Mexican American Women." *Alcohol Health and Research World* 15, no. 3: 234–38.

———. 1987. "Alcohol Consumption Patterns in Immigrant and Later Generation Mexican American Women." *Hispanic Journal of Behavioral Sciences* 9, no. 3: 299–313.

Ginzberg, Eli. 1991. "Access to Health Care for Hispanics." *Journal of the American Medical Association* 265, no. 2: 238–41.

Goldsmith, Marsha F. 1993. "Hispanic/Latino Health Issues Explored." *Journal of the American Medical Association* 269, no. 13: 1603.

———. 1990. "Forum Focuses on Hispanic-American Health." *Journal of the American Medical Association* 263, no. 5: 622.

Gonzalez, Rose I., Malika B. Gooden, and Cornelia P. Porter. 2000. "Eliminating Racial and Ethnic Disparities in Health Care." *American Journal of Nursing* 100, no. 3: 56–64.

Gonzalez-Lee, Teresa, and Harold J. Simon. 1990. *Medical Spanish: Interviewing the Latino Patient: A Cross-Cultural Perspective.* Upper Saddle River, NJ: Prentice-Hall.

Grieko, Elizabeth M., and Rachel C. Cassidy. 2001. "Overview of Race and Hispanic Origin." U.S. Census 2000 Brief, issued March 2001. C2KBR/01-1.

Guendelman, Sylvia. 1998. "Health and Disease among Hispanics." In *Handbook of Immigrant Health*, edited by S. Loue. New York: Plenum Press.

Guzmán, Betsy. 2001. "The Hispanic Population." U.S. Census 200 Brief, issued May 2001. C2KBR/01-3.

Hamilton, Nora, and Norma Stolz Chinchilla. 1991. "Central American Migration: A Framework for Analysis." *Latin American Research Review* 26, no. 1: 75–111.

Hayes-Bautista, David E. 1997. *The Health Status of Latinos in California*. The California Endowment and The California Healthcare Foundation.

Hayes-Bautista, David E., Paul Hsu, Robert Beltran, and Juan Villagomez. 1999. "The Latino Physician Shortage in California 1999." Center for the Study of Latino Health, UCLA School of Medicine.

Herrera, Carlos R., Michael P. Stern, David Goff, Evangelina Villagomez, Ariel Pablos-Mendez, Richard Scribner, Paul Sorlie, Eric Backlund, and Norman J. Johnson. 1994. "Mortality among Hispanics." *Journal of the American Medical Association* 271, no. 16: 1237–40.

Hogan-Garcia, Mikel. 1999. *The Four Skills of Cultural Diversity Competence*. Pacific Grove: Brooks/Cole.

Hondagneu-Sotelo, Pierrette. 1994. *Gendered Transitions, Mexican Experiences of Immigration*. Berkeley: University of California Press.

Hornberger, John, Haruka Itakura, and Sandra R. Wilson. 1997. "Bridging Language and Cultural Barriers between Physicians and Patients." *Public Health Reports* 12: 410–17.

Horowitz, Ruth. 1993. "The Power of Ritual in a Chicano Community: A Young Woman's Status and Expanding Family Ties." *Marriage and Family Review* 19, nos. 3–4: 257–81.

Humphry, Joseph, Lolani M. Jameson, and Sheila Beckham. 1997. "Overcoming Social and Cultural Barriers to Care for Patients with Diabetes." *Western Journal of Medicine* 167: 138–44.

Hurtado, Aida. 1995. "Variations, Combinations, and Evolutions, Latino Families in the United States." In *Understanding Latino Families: Scholarship, Policy, and Practice,* edited by R. E. Zambrana. Thousand Oaks, CA: Sage Publications.

Johnson, Elaine M., and Jane L. Delgado. 1989. "Reaching Hispanics with Messages to Prevent Alcohol and Other Drug Abuse." *Public Health Reports* 104, no. 6: 588–95.

Kaiser Permanente. 1996. *A Provider's Handbook on Culturally Competent Care, Latino Population.* The Kaiser Permanente National Diversity Council.

Karno, Marvin, and Robert B. Edgerton. 1969. "Perception of Mental Illness in a Mexican American Community." *Archives of General Psychiatry* 29: 233–38.

Kent, Mary M. 1997. *Generations of Diversity: Latinos in the United States.* Washington, DC: Population Reference Bureau.

Kikoski, John F., and Catherine K. Kikoski. 1996. *Reflexive Communication in the Culturally Diverse Workplace.* Westport, CT: Quorum Books.

Lecca, Pedro J., Ivan Quervalu, Joao V. Nunes, and Hector Gonzalez. 1998. *Cultural Competency in Health, Social, and Human Services, Directions for the Twenty-First Century.* New York: Garland Publishing.

Leininger, Madeleine. 1995. *Transcultural Nursing: Concepts, Theories, Research, and Practice.* Columbus, OH: McGraw-Hill and Greyden Press.

Leslie, Leigh A. 1993. "Families Fleeing War: The Case of Central Americans." *Marriage and Family Review* 19, nos. 1–2: 193–206.

Levene, Ricardo. 1937. *A History of Argentina.* Translated and edited by William Spence Robertson. Chapel Hill: The University of North Carolina Press. Series: The Inter-American Historical series, edited by J. A. Robertson.

Liao, Youlian, Richard S. Cooper, Guichan Cao, Ramon Durazo-Arvizu, Jay S. Kaufman, Amy Luke, and Daniel L. McGee. 1998. "Mortality Patterns among Adult Hispanics: Findings from the NHIS, 1986 to 1990. (National Health Interview Survey) *American Journal of Public Health* 88, no. 2: 227–33.

Lum, Doman. 1999. *Culturally Competent Practice.* Pacific Grove: Brooks/Cole.

Macklin, June. 1980. "All the Good and Bad in this World: Women, Traditional Medicine, and Mexican American Culture." In *Twice a Minority, Mexican American Women,* edited by M. Melville, 127–54. St. Louis: The C. V. Mosby Company.

Madriz, Esther I. 1998. "Using Focus Groups with Lower Socioeconomic Status Latina Women." *Qualitative Inquiry* 4, no. 1: 114–29.

Magaña, Aizita, and Noreen M. Clark. 1995. "Examining a Paradox: Does Religiosity Contribute to Positive Birth Outcomes in Mexican American Populations?" *Health Education Quarterly* 22, no. 1: 96–109.

Manzanedo, Hector G., Esperanza G. Walters, and Kate
    R. Lorig. 1980. "Health and Illness Perceptions of
    the Chicana." In *Twice a Minority, Mexican American
    Women*, edited by M. Melville, 191–207. St. Louis:
    The C. V. Mosby Company.
Marin, Barbara Van Oss, Eliseo J. Perez-Stable, Gerardo
    Marin, Fabio Sabogal, and Regina Otero-Sabogal.
    1990. "Attitudes and Behaviors of Hispanic Smok-
    ers: Implications for Cessation Interventions." *Health
    Education Quarterly* 17, no. 3: 287–97.
Marin, Gerardo. 1996. "Perceptions by Hispanics of Chan-
    nels and Sources of Health Messages Regarding
    Cigarette Smoking." *Tobacco Control* 5, no. 1: 30–
    36.
Marin, Gerardo, and Samuel F. Posner. 1995. "The Role of
    Gender and Acculturation on Determining the Con-
    sumption of Alcoholic Beverages among Mexican-
    Americans and Central Americans in the United
    States." *International Journal of the Addictions*, no. 7 (30
    May): 779–94.
Marin, Gerardo, and Barbara Van Oss Marin. 1991. *Research
    with Hispanic Populations*. Applied Social Research
    Methods series, volume 23. Thousand Oaks, CA:
    Sage Publications.
Markides, Kyriakos S., and Jeannine Coreil. 1986. "The
    Health of Hispanics in the Southwestern United
    States: An Epidemiologic Paradox." *Public Health
    Reports* 101, no. 3: 253–62.
Martinez, Rebeca G., Leo R. Chavez, and F. Allan Hubbell.
    1997. "Purity and Passion: Risk and Morality in
    Latina Immigrants' and Physicians' Beliefs about
    Cervical Cancer." *Medical Anthropology* 17, no. 4:
    337–62.

Mayo, Yolanda. 1997. "Machismo, Fatherhood and the Latino Family: Understanding the Concept." *Journal of Multicultural Social Work* 5, no. 1–2: 49–61.

Molina, Carlos, and Marilyn Aguirre-Molina, eds. 1994. *Latino Health in the U.S.: A Growing Challenge.* Washington, DC: American Public Health Association.

Morbidity and Mortality Weekly Report. 1999. "Self-Reported Prevalence of Diabetes among Hispanics—United States, 1994–1997." 5, no. 1: 8.

Moreno, Carmen, Matilda Alvarado, Hector Balcazar, Claire Lane, Eileen Newman, Gloria Ortiz, and Maxine Forrest. 1997. "Heart Disease Education and Prevention Program Targeting Immigrant Latinos: Using Focus Group Responses to Develop Effective Interventions." *Journal of Community Health* 22, no. 6: 435–51.

Muñoz, Eric. 1988. "Care for the Hispanic Poor: A Growing Segment of American Society." *Journal of the American Medical Association* 260, no. 18: 2711–712.

National Council of La Raza. 2001. "Policy and Programs, Health." http://www.nclr.org/policy/health.html

New York Task Force on Immigrant Health. 1996a. "Health Beliefs and Practices of Mexican Immigrants." New York University School of Medicine.

New York Task Force on Immigrant Health. 1996b. "Health Beliefs and Practices of Puerto Rican Immigrants." New York University School of Medicine.

Office of Management and Budget. 1997. "Recommendations from the Interagency Committee for the Review of the Racial and Ethnic Standards to the Office of Management and Budget Concerning Changes to the Standards for the Classification of Federal Data on Race and Ethnicity." Federal Register 7/9/97, Part II, 36873–946.

Office of Minority Health. 2000. "Assuring Cultural Competence in Health Care: Recommendations for National Standards and an Outcomes-Focused Research Agenda." Federal Register 12/22/00, 80865–79.

One America: The President's Initiative on Race. 1998. Washington, DC: The Advisory Board's Report.

Otero-Sabogal, Regina, Fabio Sabogal, Eliseo J. Perez-Stable, and Robert A. Hiatt. 1995. "Dietary Practices, Alcohol Consumption, and Smoking Behavior: Ethnic, Sex, and Acculturation Differences." Journal of the National Cancer Institute. Monographs, no. 18: 73–82.

Pablos-Mendez, Ariel. 1994. Letter to the Editor. Journal of the American Medical Association 272: 1237–38.

Padilla, Amado, ed. 1980. Acculturation: Theory, Models, and Some New Findings. Boulder, CO: Westview Press.

Palinkas, Lawrence A. 1994. "Cigarette Smoking Behavior and Beliefs of Hispanics in California." Journal of the American Medical Association 271, no. 8: 570E.

Pan American Health Organization. 2000. Annual Report of the Director. Pan American Health Organization/World Health Organization.

Pan American Health Organization. 1998. "A presentation from the Emergency Preparedness Program. Supply Management after disasters. SUMA.

Perez-Stable, Eliseo J., Gerardo Marin, and Samuel F. Posner. 1998. "Ethnic Comparison of Attitudes and Beliefs about Cigarette Smoking." Journal of General Internal Medicine 13, no. 3: 167–74.

Phillips, Kathryn A. 2000. "Barriers to Care among Racial Ethnic Groups Under Managed Care." Health Affairs 19, no. 4: 65–75.

Plante, Thomas G., Gerdinio M. Manuel, Ana V. Menendez, and David Marcotte. 1995. "Coping with Stress among Salvadoran Immigrants." *Hispanic Journal of Behavioral Sciences* 17, no. 4: 471–79.

Quinn, Michael T., and Wylie L. McNabb. 1999. "Diabetes in Hispanics: Home-based Risk Factor Reduction." *Diabetes* 48, no. 5, SA463.

Ramirez, Amelie, and Miguel Baraona. 1997. *Developing Effective Messages and Materials for Hispanic/Latino Audiences.* Technical Assistance Bulletin. Washington, DC: Center for Substance Abuse and Prevention.

Ramirez, Amelie, Roberto Villarreal, Lucina Suarez, and Estevan T. Flores. 1995. "The Emerging Hispanic Population: A Foundation for Cancer Prevention and Control." *Journal of the National Cancer Institute.* Monograph, no. 18.

Ramirez, Amelie, and Alfred L. McAlister. 1988. "Mass Media Campaign—A su salud." *Preventive Medicine* 17: 608–21.

Repak, Terry A. 1994. "Labor Market Incorporation of Central American Immigrants in Washington, DC." *Social Problems* 41, no. 1: 115–28.

Rogler, Lloyd H., Dharma E. Cortes, and Roberto G. Malgady. 1991. "Acculturation and Mental Health Status among Hispanics." *American Psychologist* 46, no. 6: 585–97.

Rueschenberg, Erich, and Raymond Buriel. 1989. "Mexican American Family Functioning and Acculturation: A Family Systems Perspective." *Hispanic Journal of Behavioral Sciences* 11, no. 3: 232–44.

Sabogal, Fabio, Regina Otero-Sabogal, Rena J. Pasick, Christopher N. H. Jenkins, and Eliseo J. Perez-Stable. 1996. "Printed Health Education Materials for Diverse Communities: Suggestions Learned from the Field." *Health Education Quarterly* 23 (supplement), S123–S141.

Sabogal, Fabio, Gerardo Marin, and Regina Otero-Sabogal. 1987. "Hispanic Familism and Acculturation: What Changes and What Doesn't?" *Hispanic Journal of Behavioral Sciences* 9, no. 4: 397–412.

Saha, Somnath, Sara H. Taggart, Miriam Komaromy, and Andrew B. Bindman. 2000. "Do Patients Choose Physicians of Their Own Race?" *Health Affairs* 19, no. 4: 76–83.

Salgado de Snyder, Nelly, Richard C. Cervantes, and Amado M. Padilla. 1990. "Migration and Post-traumatic Stress Disorders: The Case of Mexicans and Central Americans in the United States." *Acta Psiquiatrica y Psicologica de America Latina* 36, nos. 3–4: 137–45.

Shai, Donna, and Ira Rosenwaike. 1987. "Mortality among Hispanics in Metropolitan Chicago: An Examination Based on Vital Statistics Data." *Journal of Chronic Diseases*, 40: 445–51.

Smart Julie, and David W. Smart. 1994. "The Rehabilitation of Hispanics Experiencing Acculturative Stress: Implications for Practice." *Journal of Rehabilitation* 60: 8–13.

Sorlie, Paul, Eric Backlund, Norman Johnson, and Eugene Rogot. 1993. "Mortality by Hispanic Status in the United States." *Journal of the American Medical Association* 270, no. 20: 2464–68.

Spector, R. E. 1996. *Cultural Diversity in Health and Illness*. Stamford, CT: Appleton and Lange.

Stoneman, Bill. 1997. "Spanish Unites Hispanic Americans." *American Demographics* 19, no. 12.

Therrien, Melissa, and Roberto Ramirez. 2000. *The Hispanic Population in the United States: March 2000, Current Population Reports*, P20-535. Washington, DC: Bureau of the Census.

Tirado, Miguel D. 1996. "Tools for Monitoring Cultural Competence in Health Care." San Francisco, CA: Latino Coalition for a Healthy California, 1535 Mission Street, San Francisco, CA 94103.

Trueba, Enrique T. 1999. *Latinos Unidos, from Cultural Diversity to the Politics of Solidarity*. Lanham, MD: Rowman and Littlefield.

Valdez, R., Burciaga, Hal Morgenstern, E. Richard Brown, Roberto Win, Chao Wang, and William Cumberland. 1993. "Insuring Latinos Against the Cost of Illness." *Journal of the American Medical Association* 269, no. 7: 889–95.

Valdez, Rodolfo A., and Venkat Narayan. 1999. "Clustering of Hypertension and Diabetes in the U.S. Whites, Blacks, and Hispanics." *Diabetes* 48, no. 5, SA15.

Vega, William. 1994. "Latino Outlook: Good Health, Uncertain Prognosis." *Annual Review of Public Health* 15: 39–67.

Wells, Kenneth B., Jacqueline M. Golding, Richard L. Hough, M. Audrey Burnam, and Marvin Karno. 1989. "Acculturation and the Probability of Use of Health Services by Mexican Americans." *Health Services Research* 24, no. 2: 237–57.

White, Sara, and Susan Maloney. 1990. "Promoting Healthy Diets and Active Lives to Hard-to-Reach Groups: Market Research Study." *Public Health Reports* 105, no. 3: 224–31.

Breinigsville, PA USA
12 October 2010
247218BV00001B/1/A